Inside MEDICAL WASHINGTON

THE GRAND ROUNDS PRESS

Inside MEDICAL WASHINGTON

JAMES H. SAMMONS, M.D.

WHITTLE DIRECT BOOKS

The Grand Rounds Press

The Grand Rounds Press presents original short books by distinguished authors on subjects of importance to the medical profession.

The series is edited and published by Whittle Books, a business unit of Whittle Communications L.P. A new book will be published approximately every three months. The series will reflect a broad spectrum of responsible opinions. In each book the opinions expressed are those of the author, not the publisher or advertiser.

I welcome your comments on this unique endeavor.

William S. Rukeyser
Editor in Chief

*I dedicate this book to my dear wife, Jo Anne,
who has heard it all before ad infinitum, ad nauseam, and
has happily put up with it for the past 20 years.*

Photographs: 1991 AMA House of Delegates meeting by David Schlabowske, page 2; James Sammons:
courtesy of the Texas Medical Association, page 6; Sammons with Philip Overton and C. Lincoln Williston:
courtesy of the Texas Medical Association, page 10; John F. Kennedy: the Bettmann Archive, page 12;
Russell B. Roth: the Bettmann Archive, page 13; Lyndon B. Johnson and Harry S Truman:
the Bettmann Archive, page 14; Ronald Reagan montage: courtesy of the American Medical Association,
page 19; Richard M. Nixon with AMA officers: courtesy of James Sammons, page 21; Jimmy Carter:
the Bettmann Archive, page 24; Otis Bowen: AP/Wide World Photos, page 25; Joseph Califano:
AP/Wide World Photos, page 26; Elliot Richardson: the Bettmann Archive, page 27; Carolyne Davis: courtesy
of Carolyne Davis, page 31; William Hsiao by Nicholas Nixon, page 33; John Sununu: ©Diana Walker/Gamma
Liaison, page 38; Richard Darman: ©Larry Downing/Gamma Liaison, page 39; Expenditure target advertise-
ment: courtesy of the American Medical Association, page 40; John D. Rockefeller IV:
©Brad Markel/Gamma Liaison, page 41; Fortney Stark: the Bettmann Archive, page 42; Medicaid patients by
Misha Erwitt/Magnum, page 48; Joseph Boyle: AP/Wide World Photos, page 53; James Tallon:
Louise Noakes, page 56; Scott Matheson:
AP/Wide World Photos, page 57.

Library of Congress Catalog Card Number: 91-66025
Sammons, James H., M.D.
Inside Medical Washington
ISBN 1-879736-03-9
ISSN 1053-6620

I offer my thanks to Richard Sorian for his assistance in researching and writing this book.

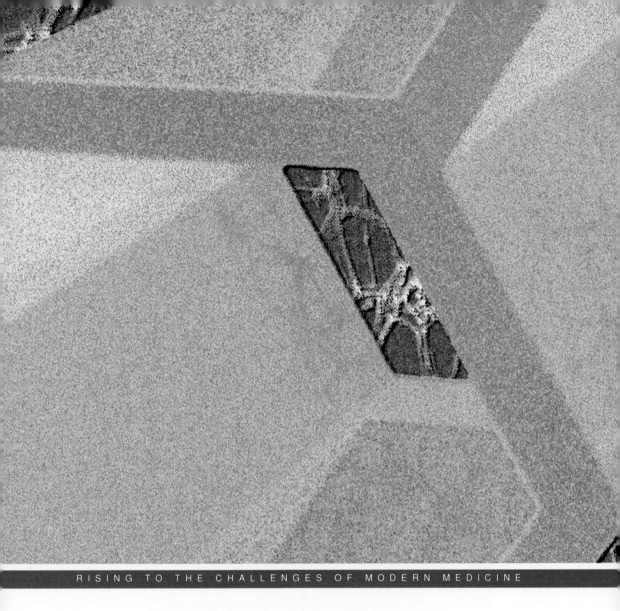

THE PRACTICE OF MEDICINE IN THE TWENTIETH CENTURY
PRESENTS A COMPLEX AND EVOLVING SERIES OF CHALLENGES.
TODAY MORE THAN EVER BEFORE, PHYSICIANS REQUIRE INNOVATIVE
THERAPEUTIC AGENTS THAT SUPPORT AND FACILITATE
THEIR ENDEAVORS. SYNTEX RESPONDS...

A

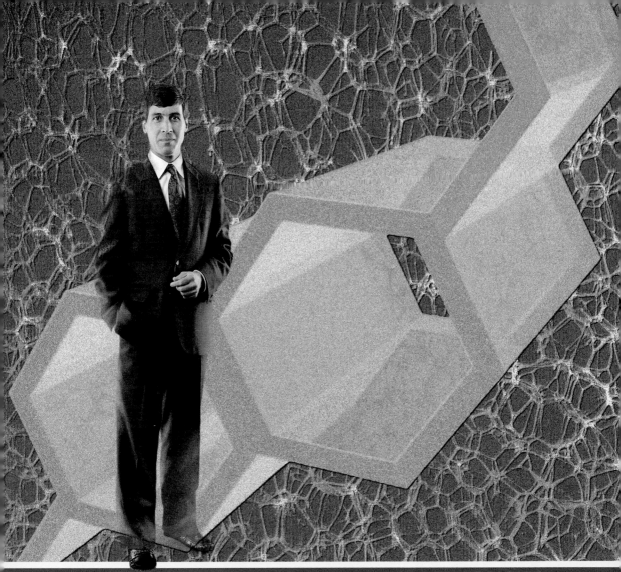

RISING TO THE CHALLENGES OF MODERN MEDICINE

At Syntex, we consider our relationship with practicing physicians to be a collaboration. They provide us with a clear understanding of the challenges of modern medicine, and we respond by pursuing new avenues of investigation that may lead to innovative pharmaceutical products. Our vision encompasses not only meeting the medical challenges of today, but also exploring the therapeutic possibilities of tomorrow.

Timothy P. Spiro, MD
Vice President
Medical Affairs Division
Syntex Laboratories, Inc.

B

PREFACE

I am convinced that the majority of physicians in this country do not understand how Washington works, or the extent to which federal legislators in Washington are involved in setting the national agenda on health affairs. Physicians need to understand the roles played by organizations like the American Medical Association and specialty societies like the American Society of Internal Medicine and the American College of Surgeons in trying to affect the course of policymaking in Washington, where we're dealing with a great many nonphysicians whose actions have a direct impact on the practice of medicine.

But the importance of this book goes well beyond the role of medical societies. This is a call to arms for American physicians to shake the dust off their boots and get involved in the political process. The federal government is determined to leave its mark on the medical profession, and in my opinion that mark will be one that will make the practice of medicine more difficult and less helpful to patients and their doctors.

All doctors in this country—no matter their political party, no matter their race, sex, or religion—ought to be involved in their local congressional elections. Physicians ought to support a candidate; they ought to be knowledgeable about that candidate's stand; they ought to have input into that candidate's platform and thinking on issues affecting health care. Too many doctors don't know their congressmen or senators, and because many have never taken the time to become involved in a campaign, their congressmen and senators don't know them either. The only way you can have productive input is to get personally involved in the political process

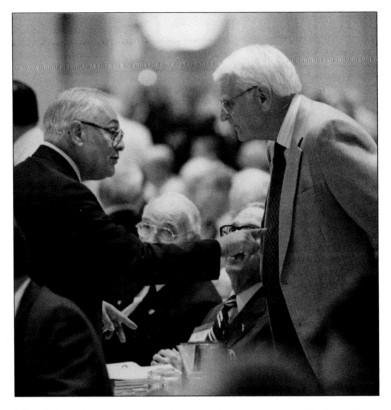

Physicians have a voice if they choose to use it. Dr. G. L. Andriole (left) and Dr. Richard McMurray use theirs at the AMA's 1991 House of Delegates meeting in Chicago.

at home. You don't have to start joining large organizations that require lots of your time. Start small: join the Rotary Club or the Kiwanis Club, or just go to your church. The important thing is to stand up and be heard.

Far too often physicians act as bystanders, watching the political process go by like a parade, criticizing the costumes of some of the participants or the way they walk but doing absolutely nothing to alter the course of that parade. Now, some doctors will say, "I'm busy. I've got a practice to run, a staff to supervise, patients to see and to treat, bills to pay, etc., etc., etc." I have one word to say to those folks: in print I'll change it to "Horsefeathers!"

You're talking to a fellow who has spent his whole life in

medical politics. Nobody's that busy. You can get involved at night, you can participate in meetings of county and state medical societies, you can get up and have your say. The thing that sets medicine apart from a host of other professions is that it is organized to ensure that physicians who want to have a say can. The opportunity is there if you'll just use it.

We can either force a change in what has become a convoluted and often misguided system, or we can live with the consequences of that system to the detriment of our patients. If enough physicians choose to get involved, then this book will have been worthwhile.

CHAPTER ONE

A GOLDEN ERA LOST

t's hard to believe sometimes that it has been nearly 40 years since I began practicing medicine back in Highlands, Texas, a small town across the San Jacinto River from Houston. When I moved there from my home in Alabama in 1952, the town only had about 3,000 people, and three doctors. I was the fourth. I was a general practitioner, serving the many needs of the people of the town for 15 years.

Although it was hard leaving my first practice and my first patients, I felt I had to move on to improve my skills as a general practitioner and to provide for my growing family. So in 1967 I left Highlands for nearby Baytown, where I built a group practice that eventually numbered 11 physicians. It was small-town medicine at its best. Having babies was still fashionable in those days, and having GPs deliver them was in fashion, too. I delivered babies in the hospital, in homes, on the floors of churches in the middle of hurricanes, in schoolhouses, and, yes, in the backs of cars and taxicabs.

It was a wonderful time to be a doctor in these United States. It was what I like to think of as the golden age of American medicine, a time when we were conquering disease and no advancement seemed out of the question or beyond our reach. When I started practicing medicine, there was no polio vaccine. My God, we had iron lungs in hospital rooms, we had iron lungs in the halls, we had little kids of all ages with polio, and we had adults who were dying from polio. I recall taking care of one family with five children, every one of whom had polio one summer. Fortunately, none of them died and none of them were in iron lungs, but that family left a lasting impression on me, a young doctor with a family of his own. I saw active typhoid cases and active diphtheria cases. You'd be hard-pressed to find a medical school graduate of the last 10 or 15 years who has ever seen one of those, and thank God that's true.

But it was an exciting time because we never believed we couldn't beat whatever we came up against. With the help of such heroes as Dr. Jonas Salk, we conquered polio and lots of other diseases that caused death or disability. As a result, medicine was regarded as a noble profession, one that the mothers and fathers of this country were proud to see their sons and daughters join.

Unfettered by regulators who told us what we could or could not do, physicians simply went out and did it. In return, our patients had a strong degree of faith in their family physicians, and that made it a sheer pleasure to be a physician. There was very little government interference in the practice of medicine, and very little interference from insurance companies.

The first fight I ever had with an insurance company was back in the mid-1950s. I was still practicing in Highlands when I got a letter from Blue Cross/Blue Shield of Texas about a pregnant patient of mine. I was sure this woman had an active duodenal ulcer that was complicating what should have been a routine pregnancy, and to confirm my diagnosis I had her X-rayed. The problem was I didn't put her in the hospital first, and at that time the Blues wouldn't pay for an X-ray unless a patient had been hospitalized for 48 hours. That made no sense to me; the woman certainly did not need to be hospitalized, and it would have been a colossal waste of money and a bed to put her there. Nevertheless, rules were rules, and the Blues weren't going to pay for that X-ray. I thought then—and I think now—that had to be the epitome of stupidity.

But the interference of the Texas Blues in the 1950s pales in comparison with what physicians face today. Back then there was no preadmission certification, no utilization-review committee, none of the hierarchical arrangements from third-party payers—the Blues, the commercial insurers, the government, HMOs, managed-care systems, whatever—that exist in medicine today. The hassles just weren't there.

I quit the active practice of medicine in 1974 and left Texas for Chicago to become executive vice-president of the American Medical Association. (In that organization, the position of EVP is similar to that of CEO in a large business.) My decision to accept the offer to head up the AMA didn't surprise a lot of people who knew me well. I had been a dues-paying member of the AMA since I entered the medical profession and had been quite active in the Texas Medical Association. In fact, I served as president of the TMA in 1971 and 1972 and had been a member of the AMA board of trustees since 1970. So agreeing to take over the AMA at a most difficult time in its history was not out of keeping with my character.

Maybe if I had known what was ahead of me, I would have stayed back in Baytown. I spent a good part of my first year working overtime to deal with the severe financial crisis facing the organization. In short order, I was faced with the difficult, painful task of firing a number of AMA employees to bring our expenses in line with our annual income. That was probably one of the toughest decisions I had to make—after all, some of those folks had families. But once the pain was over with, we started rebuilding the AMA so that it could adequately represent the half-million physicians who depended on it for continuing education and for representation in Washington. Within a couple of years, we had grown so much we were able to expand our staff beyond the size it was when I took over.

I spent much of the next 15 years fighting against the kind of mindless bureaucracy demonstrated by the Texas Blues back in the 1950s. Since I moved to Chicago, I've heard more horror stories about the practice of medicine than I guess I knew existed in the 22 years I was practicing. We at the AMA and our colleagues in the national specialty groups worked hard to overcome these obstacles and to convince senators, congressmen, and presidents that they were doing more to handicap medicine than they were doing to help the people they claimed to represent.

Now, no one likes to admit failure—I certainly don't—but looking at the state of medicine today and the inability of many people, particularly poor families, to gain access to what is still

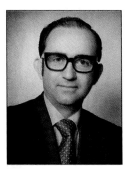

Dr. Sammons in 1974, shortly before he left Texas to become executive vice-president of the American Medical Association

CHALLENGE:

TO BRING INTO FOCUS THE POWER OF THE FIRST INJECTABLE ANALGESIC NSAID. SYNTEX RESPONDS…

SYNTEX

C

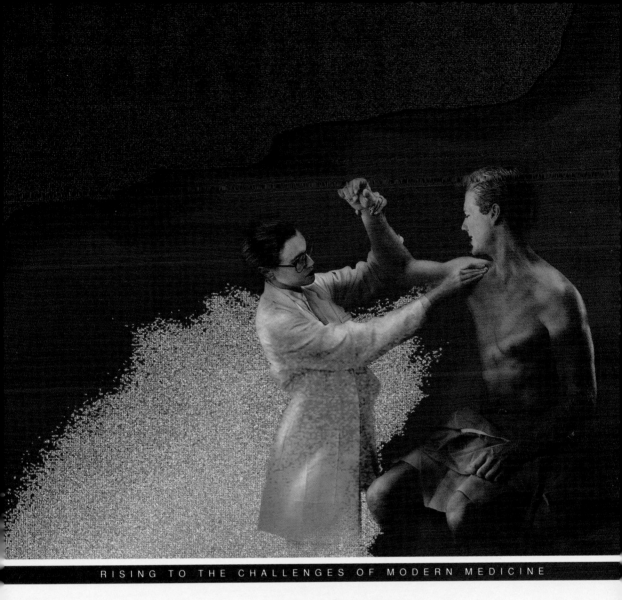

RISING TO THE CHALLENGES OF MODERN MEDICINE

TORADOL® IM
(KETOROLAC TROMETHAMINE) 15, 30, 60 MG.

OUR DEVELOPMENT OF THE FIRST <u>INJECTABLE ANALGESIC</u> NSAID BRINGS
YET ANOTHER BREAKTHROUGH AGENT TO THE SYNTEX THERAPEUTIC LINE.
INDICATED FOR THE SHORT-TERM MANAGEMENT OF PAIN,
TORADOL™ PROVIDES NARCOTIC STRENGTH
WITHOUT NARCOTIC COMPLICATIONS.

AS WITH OTHER NONSTEROIDAL DRUGS,
THE MOST FREQUENTLY REPORTED SIDE EFFECTS ARE GASTROINTESTINAL,
WITH SOME GI SYMPTOMS REPORTED BY 3% TO 9% OF PATIENTS
IN CLINICAL TRIALS. SEE "WARNINGS," "PRECAUTIONS," AND "ADVERSE REACTIONS"
SECTIONS OF COMPLETE PRESCRIBING INFORMATION
ON PAGES XVII-XX OF THE APPENDIX.

D

the greatest health-care system in the world, I have to say we failed to influence enough of those policymakers. But things would be a lot worse if we hadn't been in there knocking heads and counting votes. Just imagine what medicine would be like today if we hadn't been able to depend on the support of hundreds of thousands of doctors across the United States to call, write, and speak to lawmakers to help convince them of the right path to take on health-care issues.

I firmly believe that if doctors hadn't been involved in the process of government, the degree of regulation in this country would be much greater than many physicians would be able to bear. Don't forget, it wasn't too long ago that people like Senator Ted Kennedy and his supporters in the labor movement believed they were poised to enact national health insurance. If you want to know what that would be like, just take a look at Great Britain, where patients must wait months for needed tests and treatments. Look at Canada, whose patients are streaming over the border to get care in U.S. facilities from American doctors.

Still, I feel strongly that something must be done, and done soon, to change the path we're going down. Medicine is no longer an enjoyable profession. In fact, I can't count the number of times I've heard from lifetime colleagues and friends that if they had it to do over they wouldn't be practicing medicine today. And a lot of them say they are telling their sons and daughters to stay out of medicine and choose another field. That makes me sad, and it makes me angry.

Washington is always looking to save money in any way it can, and in the process, government is imposing so much red tape and bureaucratic nonsense on physicians that it seems like a doctor today can't make a move without four or five bureaucrats looking over his shoulder. And all of this regulation hasn't brought about any improvement in the practice of medicine or the state of the nation's health. Today more than 30 million of our citizens are without health insurance, and millions more have barely enough coverage to pay for a major catastrophe. Working men and women often must choose between taking their child to a doctor and paying the monthly mortgage.

But I've always believed it's much easier to be against something than it is to be for something, and I am convinced that being for something is the only way to make progress. That's why during my time at the AMA and today as a private citizen I have always looked for answers to the problems confronting medicine and the people it serves. In the following chapters, I intend to lay out a series of choices for the nation and suggest a course that I believe will bring us closer to what I think we all want: access for the maximum number of people to an affordable and high-quality system of medical care that encourages innovation and progress and doesn't stymie the entrepreneurial spirit of the men and women who choose medicine for a career.

I believe we are at a rare moment when we can influence the health of the next generation with the decisions we make today. If we make the right choices, we can ensure a longer and healthier life for our people. But if we make the wrong choices, we will continue to drive good people from the medical profession and harm the patients they would have served.

CHAPTER TWO

THE MEDICARE MESS

major contributing factor to the decline of American medicine in recent years has been intrusion by the federal government, which decided to get involved in financing medical care in 1965 with the enactment of Medicare and Medicaid. Since then, the bureaucrats in Washington have become a third party in the doctor-patient relationship—most times, an unwelcome one.

The national Democratic Party's push to create a federal program of health-insurance coverage for everyone who reaches the age of 65 started in earnest during President Harry Truman's administration in the late 1940s, and continued through the Eisenhower and Kennedy administrations in the '50s and '60s. Many of us, myself included, never agreed with the Medicare program as it was proposed. We felt the government was making a promise it could not keep and was offering a single level of insurance to millions of people regardless of their needs and their ability to pay.

Organized medicine took some pretty big hits in the media and in Washington for this opposition. People said we didn't care about the needs of our patients, that all we cared about was our wallets. Well, I said then, and I say now, that is just rubbish. We fought against Medicare as it was proposed because we did care about our patients and we worried what would become of them if the government got into the business of providing medical care.

So we did everything we could to make sure it didn't hap-

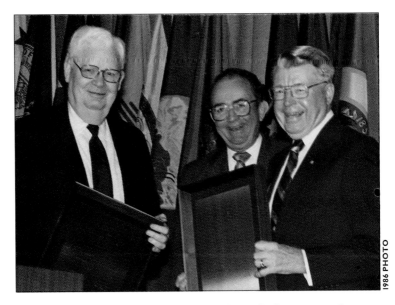

1986 PHOTO

Dr. Sammons with Texas Medical Association general counsel Philip R. Overton (left) and executive secretary C. Lincoln Williston (right), who in 1962 helped TMA form TexPAC.

pen. In 1961, the AMA, hoping to further involve physicians in the political process, created the American Medical Political Action Committee—AMPAC—to raise money for contributions to candidates for Congress. Meanwhile, some of the states, including Texas, California, and Illinois, had already created state PACs. They didn't call them PACs in those days, but that's what they were.

In Texas, in the 1950s, we had an informal group of people that got together two or three times a year. It included Philip R. Overton, who was general counsel of the Texas Medical Association; C. Lincoln Williston, executive secretary of the TMA; and whoever was the president of the organization that particular year. We sat around the table and talked about the need to raise money to support political candidates. The way to do that in those days was to reach in your pocket and simply put your pro rata share into the pot. And that's what we did.

Because the political climate wasn't right, Truman wasn't able to get much support for his Medicare proposal. The issue remained dormant for most of the 1950s—President Dwight D. Eisenhower was opposed to involving the government in the business of providing health care. But the Democratic Congress continued to push the idea; in 1958, a young senator named John F. Kennedy got a Medicare bill through the Senate knowing full well that Eisenhower would veto it. The bill never made it out of the House, but Kennedy had an issue for his 1960 campaign for president.

During that campaign, Kennedy made it clear that, if elected, he would push for Medicare. That helped energize senior citizens, who turned out in droves to vote for the Democratic candidate. And when Kennedy beat Richard Nixon by a narrow 114,000-vote margin, many credited the victory to the support of those elderly voters.

Kennedy didn't forget it. Once inaugurated, he began pressing for a Medicare program that would pay for 90 days of hospitalization each year for all citizens over age 64, and he made a dramatic speech in favor of the proposal at New York's Madison Square Garden in 1962. But the new president didn't have much support from the majority in Congress: the conservative Southern Democrats wanted no part of a new government health-care program. We in organized medicine predicted that the cost of Kennedy's Medicare proposal would far exceed the estimates of his administration and the bean counters up on Capitol Hill. By the time Kennedy was assassinated in 1963, his Medicare plan was going nowhere.

But John F. Kennedy's death was a tragedy for the nation, and it convinced a lot of people that they had to complete his unfinished agenda. One of the items on that agenda was Medicare.

Lyndon B. Johnson, the new president, also was a strong supporter of Medicare (he had helped Kennedy push his bill through the Senate back in 1958), and the Medicare bill really got rolling after Johnson was reelected in 1964 by a landslide over Barry Goldwater. That victory also swept in a tremendous pro-Johnson majority in both the House and the Senate, and Johnson promised to use his mandate to create what he called the Great Society. Included in that was Medicare.

The Medicare concept—taking care of the elderly who cannot take care of themselves—is not wrong. What is wrong

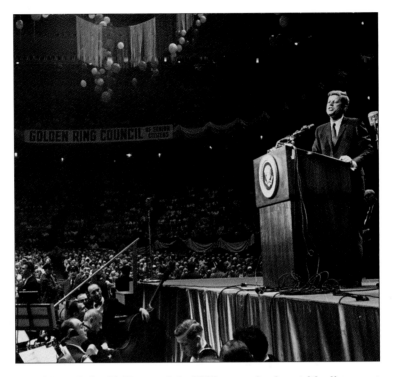

President John F. Kennedy's 1962 speech about Medicare at Madison Square Garden didn't win points from organized medicine, but it galvanized popular support for the program.

is the assumption that the entire over-65 population is incapable of making decisions, incapable of taking care of itself, and incapable of paying a part of its own health-care costs. People on the lower end of the income scale have always had a problem paying premiums, paying the deductibles, and paying the coinsurance. The ones on the upper end of the income scale have never had a problem with that, and they've freeloaded. They're still freeloading.

Organized medicine recognized the need of many of the elderly—particularly the poor—to get assistance with their medical bills, and in 1965 we came forward with a proposal we called Eldercare. It was the idea of Dr. Russell B. Roth, an Erie, Pennsylvania, urologist who later became president of the AMA. Not only would Eldercare have underwritten premiums for hospitalization insurance for those who needed financial help, it also would have paid physicians' bills and the cost of other outpatient care. It would not have paid bills for those people who could afford to purchase their own insurance.

Eldercare was a good program, but it was too little and too late. The Medicare steamroller was already rolling down the hill at a hundred miles an hour, and there wasn't anything that anybody was going to do to stop it. The best we could hope for was that somehow or other we could change its direction.

With Lyndon Johnson, organized medicine was up against one of the best politicians of his time. Johnson knew what he wanted, and no one was going to stop him. Our attempts to defeat Medicare were weakened by the support Johnson got from the hospital industry. Some of the state hospital associations joined the parade because Johnson and his people told them, "We're going to take care of the hospitals by providing cost-plus reimbursement." That meant the government would pay all of the costs of a hospital stay for a Medicare patient and then add 2 percent pure profit. It was no wonder that some of the hospital associations in this country, including the Texas Hospital Association, jumped on the Medicare bandwagon. But that created some schisms between physicians and hospital administrators that lasted for damn near 20 years.

Blaming hospital administrators or Lyndon Johnson for the problems caused by Medicare isn't totally fair: doctors were part of their own ruination. Johnson's original Medicare proposal did not include physicians; he only wanted to pay for 60 days of hospital care. If we had been as smart in the 1960s as we are in the 1990s, we'd still be outside the program. But the medical profession decided that it wanted to be in, and there's no doubt in my mind that medicine generated its own difficulties when it demanded to be included. There is also no doubt in my mind that those in medicine who made that decision made it with total honesty and integrity. They were not looking at the dollars and cents of it; they were looking at the need to take care of people, many of whom had not had access to primary care before.

And Johnson himself was determined to get physicians into his corner. Just before the Medicare program was passed by Congress, President Johnson and Wilbur Cohen, an undersecretary of HEW, met with a group of AMA leaders at the

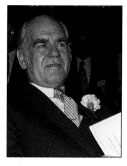

Dr. Russell B. Roth, an Erie, Pennsylvania, urologist, conceived the Eldercare plan, which the AMA proposed in 1965 as an alternative to Medicare.

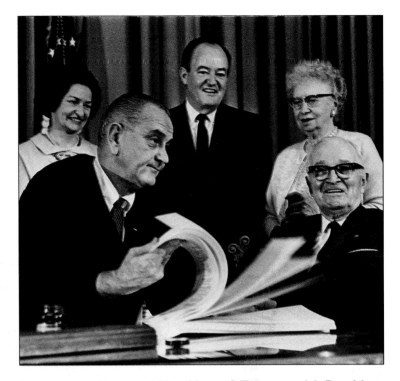

Former president and Mrs. Harry S Truman with President and Mrs. Lyndon B. Johnson at the 1965 signing of the Medicare bill. With them is Vice-President Hubert Humphrey.

White House in a last-ditch effort to work out a deal. They went through some 21 things that the AMA was objecting to. And Johnson told Cohen, "Fix it. If that's their problem, fix it."

Cohen told me that story years later. In fact, he used to come and see me in Chicago in the last few years before he died, and he had changed some of his basic thoughts about the Medicare program. He was beginning to have concerns that some of the rest of us had had for a long time. He used to say, "I wish now that I had listened to you guys. We could have put a different twist on this and gotten some more of the private sector in it."

Few people realize that Medicare could have jeopardized the health-insurance industry. The final legislation effectively rendered all private policies covering people over age 65 null and void. But Johnson and Cohen were smart. They knew they needed the support of the insurers if Medicare was going to fly in Congress, so they allowed them to become the fiscal intermediaries for the program. Today, that's a multibillion-dollar program, and the profits go right into the pockets of private insurers. Like the move to provide cost-plus reimbursement to hospitals, the change Johnson and Cohen made in their bill bought the support of the insurance industry and made defeating the bill that much more difficult.

The Medicare program sailed right through. Johnson was in his Great Society, the great catharsis of the American people following John Kennedy's assassination. In the first thousand days of Johnson's administration we passed more social legislation than we had since 1935, and more than has ever been passed in a comparable time since.

Medicare went into effect in 1966. In the early days, things weren't so bad. The paperwork wasn't all that difficult. You had to run everybody—including doctors—through the process of training. Some of us had a leg up on the paperwork because we'd been working with the military medical program that is now called CHAMPUS. In my part of southeast Texas (the whole Houston-Galveston area), there were a whole lot of military folks, both retirees and actives and their dependents, and all of us had gotten very well acquainted with the Defense Department's health-care program. And when NASA moved into the area in the 1960s and built the space center down in Clear Lake Shores, we had more and more people. So the Medicare program wasn't all that new, nor was it that complicated.

But as the years went by, the government heaped more and more regulation on the profession and on the patients. Today, a doctor can't do hardly a thing without some insurer or bureaucrat breathing down his neck.

The government is not totally to blame for this. Some of my colleagues in the medical profession have taken advantage of Medicare and have caused most of the problems that the vast majority of physicians in this country do not deserve to have. This greedy little group has misused the program. I've seen avarice, substandard medicine, manufactured illnesses, bill-padding—I've seen all the things that everybody knows happen. A very, very small percentage of the physicians in this country have done any of that, but in the process, those physicians have made it nearly impossible for the vast majority of honest and caring doctors to take care of their patients without all this intervention.

Now, Medicare has done essentially what the planners said it would do. It has indeed provided medical care for millions and millions of people over the age of 65. Where I argue with it is where it provides the same benefits and the same premiums, deductibles, and coinsurance for the upper end of the income scale as for the lower end of the income scale. Today, people at the lower end are still disadvantaged, and the upper end is still freeloading.

CHAPTER THREE

MISADVENTURES IN DEMOCRACY

espite medicine's concerns about the enactment of Medicare in 1965, the program got off the ground pretty well and seemed to be working. But no sooner had it gone into effect than the bureaucrats in Washington started looking for ways to cut costs. As we predicted, the government began to take advantage of its new role as payer for health-care services by imposing itself on the doctor-patient relationship in the name of cost containment.

From day one, Medicare lived beyond its means. The estimates by the authors of the legislation that Medicare would cost $4 billion by 1970 proved to be a lot of hogwash. The actual cost was close to $7 billion. When Medicare started, working Americans were asked to pay a tax of 0.35 percent on the first $6,600 they earned each year to pay for Part A coverage. By 1970, Congress had increased that tax twice, to 0.60 percent of $7,800.

The first big round of cost-cutting measures for the medical profession came in 1972 with the imposition of the professional standards review organizations, or PSROs. These local groups were supposedly created to assure a high quality of medical care and lower costs for senior citizens on Medicare and for the indigent on Medicaid. But all they were really concerned with was costs. They hassled and harangued doctors and hospitals and attempted to place themselves between the practitioners of medicine and their patients.

The AMA fought hard against the creation of PSROs in 1972 and continued to fight against the regulations once they were in place. It took us 10 years, but finally, in 1982, Congress agreed to repeal the PSRO program and disassemble the nearly 200 local organizations it had created. However, in place of PSROs, Congress established a new program known as peer review organizations, or PROs. These 54 statewide organizations were given many of the same tasks as the PSROs and powers to recommend penalties for physicians they believed had violated a standard of practice. The medical community has had many problems with the PROs—in fact, one of my longtime colleagues says the only difference between PSROs and PROs is they took the "standards" out.

But by the 1980s, the country and organized medicine were dealing with a much larger problem than the PSROs. The inflationary decade of the 1970s (caused in many ways by such grand schemes as Medicare) had left the national economy in ruins. The country faced double-digit inflation and double-digit interest rates. For many Americans, the idea of being able to afford a home was becoming obsolete. The state of the economy—along with the hostage situation in Iran—helped elect Ronald Reagan president in 1980.

The vast majority of physicians were big supporters of Ronald Reagan. He had been a friend of medicine in the early 1960s—in fact, he had worked with the AMA to try to defeat Medicare and pass our Eldercare proposal. In his two terms as governor of California, however, we in organized medicine had a somewhat uneven relationship with Reagan.

Now, granted, most of the problems that California physicians had with the Reagan administration had little to do with the governor. The real problem was with Reagan's health secretary, Dr. Earl Brian. Brian was a brilliant person, but his management style was atrocious. He would make up his mind what he wanted to do on a health-policy issue and then call in members of the professional community to get their advice. If they agreed with him, everything was fine. But if they disagreed, he would just ignore them.

We had heard some rumors that if Reagan was elected in 1980, Earl Brian stood a good chance of being named secretary of the Department of Health and Human Services. I knew

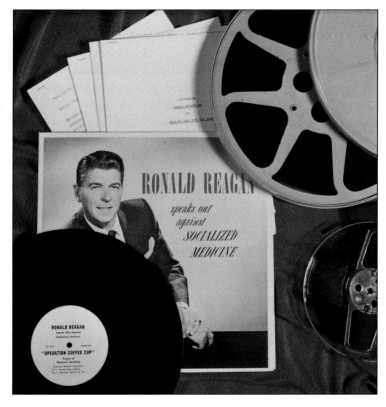

Ronald Reagan was a spokesman for organized medicine in the early 1960s, but as president, he imposed some of the toughest cost-cutting measures ever on U.S. physicians.

that if that came to pass, the doctors in California would just go up the wall.

Before Reagan was elected, a delegation from the AMA that included myself, our president, Joe Boyle, and my top aide, Joe Miller, met with Reagan out in California. I said to him, "Governor, you're running and doctors in this country are basically a conservative group of people. They've known you for years, not only in the motion picture and television industries, but also as you traveled around the country for General Electric. But what doctors don't understand is why the doctors in California have had such an incredible problem with you as governor."

Well, Reagan looked at me like I'd absolutely lost my mind.

He said, "Why, I haven't had any problem with the doctors in California. I'm the best friend they've ever had."

At that point I thought Joe Boyle was going to go right through the ceiling. You see, Joe was a practicing physician in California and a past president of the CMA. Joe said, "Governor, what Dr. Sammons told you is absolutely right. We've had more trouble with you than with any other governor."

Again, Reagan looked at both of us like we'd lost our marbles. He said, "Why, I just can't believe it. I've had no problems with the doctors."

Fortunately Ed Meese, who was Reagan's campaign manager and had been his chief of staff in California, turned around to him and said, "Governor, there was a problem— there were several problems. We took care of the problems for you, but yes, there were problems." And Reagan looked at him like he'd lost his marbles, too. He said, "Ed, I've never heard that before."

We made our feelings about Earl Brian pretty clear at that meeting. No promises were made—in fact, Reagan's aides said they didn't even have a long list of candidates for any of the cabinet jobs. Once he was elected, of course, Reagan chose former Pennsylvania senator Richard Schweiker to head HHS. Brian never did get a job in the Reagan administration.

But that incident was just a small indication of what we would learn to expect from Reagan. Most of the time in Washington you deal with a president's staff, and we got along very well with the Reagan staff. In fact, of all the presidents I've dealt with, his staff was probably the best. But every once in a while, there comes a time when you want to meet with the Big Guy.

Now, there are two ways you meet with a president. There are small meetings—just you and maybe one top lieutenant with the president and one or two of his staff members in the Oval Office. Then there are big meetings, where you've got a team of people and the president has a team, and you usually meet in the Cabinet Room at the White House. We met twice with Reagan at the White House, but it was never in the Oval Office. It was always in the Cabinet Room because he always had a large retinue. In these kinds of meetings, you deal with the president in a very straightforward and abbreviated way. You're always very limited in the length of time you can stay

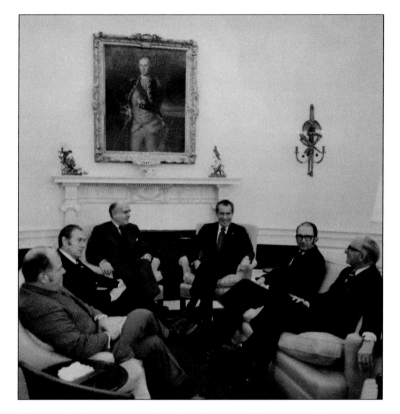

Richard Nixon in the Oval Office in 1973 with AMA executives (left to right) Joe D. Miller, Dr. Malcolm C. Todd, Dr. Russell B. Roth, Dr. Sammons, and Dr. Ernest B. Howard

with him, and you can't get in to see him as often as you'd like.

The first time we met with Reagan after he was elected, we wanted to find out if he intended to follow up on his campaign promise to physicians to create a separate Department of Health. Since the mid-1950s, federal health-care policy had been the responsibility of a larger department that dealt with many other issues. Until 1980, it was part of the Department of Health, Education, and Welfare (HEW). A separate Department of Education was created in 1980, and the remainder of HEW was renamed the Department of Health and Human Services (HHS). The AMA believed that creating a separate Department of Health would focus much-needed government attention on health-care matters. And we wanted a law that required the head of that department to be a physician.

We weren't asking for much. After all, many states already had separate health departments, and they often required the top person to be a physician. And during his campaign Reagan had promised to back our proposal. But when we met with him, nothing had been done.

We said, "Mr. President, during the campaign you promised that you were going to support a separate secretary of health, but nothing has happened."

Reagan turned to his entourage and said, "Make it happen. I keep my promises." His staff said, "Yes, Mr. President." And we all walked out of the room. I don't know what happened to that order, but I can tell you for damn sure nothing happened.

The second time we went in, we said, "Mr. President, you know you gave the order to create a secretary for health, and nothing has happened." Reagan said, "I did, didn't I?" And again, he said to his staff, "Make it happen." Again, nothing happened.

Later, the president came to an AMA meeting and some of us sat down and had lunch with him. He told some great stories about his broadcasting years and his movie years. Finally I said to him, "Mr. President, we're running out of time. For the third time, we want a separate secretary of health." He said, "It's going to happen."

It still ain't happened.

I've met with half a dozen presidents during my career, and they're all different. The two most accessible presidents I've known were Richard Nixon and Gerald Ford. We didn't always see eye-to-eye with them, but neither one ever refused us an invitation to meet.

Both Nixon and Ford had worked closely with us before they became president. When he was in the Senate and when he was Eisenhower's vice-president, Nixon had quite a few dealings with physicians and their representatives about issues of interest to the physicians of California and of the country as a whole. And Nixon relied on physician groups for advice on his health-care platform during his 1968 presidential campaign. Hubert Humphrey, his Democratic opponent, was promising

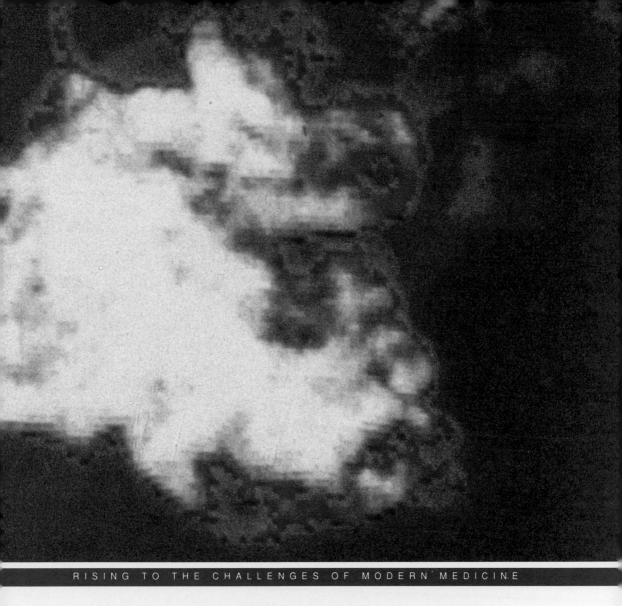

Challenge:

To address the devastation of stroke. Syntex responds...

 SYNTEX

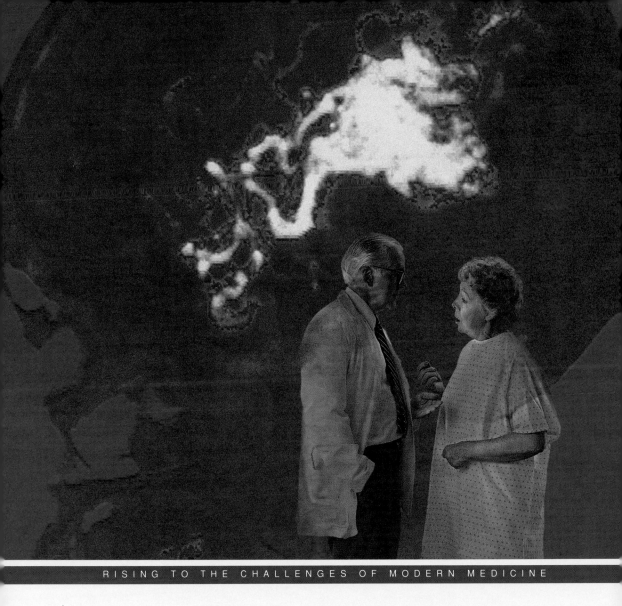

WE ARE INVESTIGATING A PROMISING COMPOUND THAT MAY REDUCE
THE RISK OF STROKE AND THE DISABILITY THAT ENSUES.

national health insurance; Nixon opposed that idea. Nixon wanted the approval of medicine; he believed in what medicine was doing. Ford had known many of us, including me, when he was in the House and serving as the Republican leader. AMPAC had worked with Ford in the 1960s to help identify candidates for the House.

Jimmy Carter was a different story. He came into the White House mad at physicians because he had been involved in a terrible fight with the Georgia Medical Association. The first time I went in to talk with him, he spent the first five minutes berating me about the treatment he had received at the hands of the Georgia Medical Association. When he finally stopped, I said, "Mr. President, you've got to understand, that's not the AMA's fault. State medical societies are all independent units. We have no control over them. It's sort of like a president and the Congress." Well, he went on for another five minutes anyway.

Carter had promised national health insurance during his campaign, and he did try to introduce such a bill. But interestingly, Carter had a harder time getting his own party to help him pass it than he did with the AMA. Ted Kennedy wouldn't hold still for President Carter's idea of introducing national health insurance gradually; Ted wanted it all at once and was willing to gamble on getting nothing. Well, nothing was what he got.

Surprisingly, Jimmy Carter has become a very good friend of the medical profession since he left the White House in 1981. He opened the Carter Presidential Center in Atlanta in 1982, and among other things, he has spent a good deal of time and energy on such issues as eliminating the Guinea worm and improving childhood-immunization programs in Africa. He's even written articles for *The Journal of the American Medical Association* and has been the recipient of some awards from organized medicine.

Most physicians were quite happy with the election of Ronald Reagan in 1980. He had promised to get the government off the backs of the people, to reduce regulation, and to eliminate waste and fraud in government programs. These were all things physicians could support.

But once he got into the White House, President Reagan

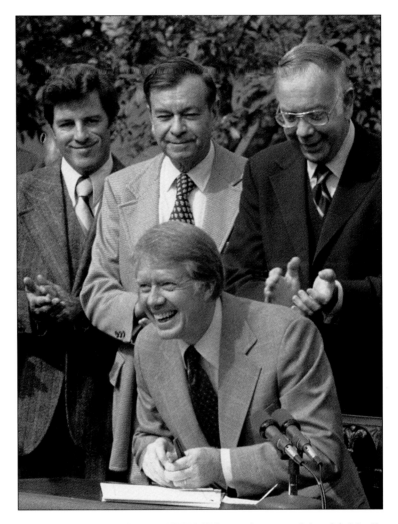

President Carter signs a 1977 bill boosting penalties for Medicare and Medicaid fraud. His relations with organized medicine, once stormy, have improved since he left office.

was a different story. Rather than reducing the amount of regulation in the health-care field, Reagan and his administration dramatically increased the red tape. By the time he left office, physicians and other health-care providers were among the most heavily regulated professions in the nation.

After our first meeting with the president-elect in 1980, we had some idea of Reagan's management style—he lived in a world of his own. I finally quit worrying about getting in to see the president because I knew it didn't make a bit of difference. In the Reagan years, the key was to get in to see his top staff. For the first term the key players included James Baker, the chief of staff; Ed Meese, the president's counselor; and Michael Deaver, the deputy chief of staff, who guarded the president's image. We could always get an answer from them—it may not have been the answer we wanted, but we could get one.

The biggest change during the Reagan years was the rise to power of the Office of Management and Budget (OMB). As the agency that controls the budget-making process, the OMB has always been important, particularly since the Nixon administration. But during Reagan's two terms, the OMB became the single most powerful agency on domestic-policy issues. Reagan had appointed David Stockman to run OMB during his first term in office, and Stockman had his fingers in everything, including health-care financing. Each of the three people who would serve as Reagan's secretaries of Health and Human Services had to bow to the wishes of Stockman or those of his successor, James Miller III.

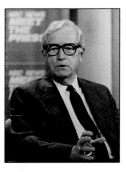

Former Indiana governor Otis Bowen, Reagan's third secretary of Health and Human Services, was the first physician to hold that post.

Things aren't any different now with President Bush. Richard Darman, who runs the OMB for Bush, has been in government for nearly 20 years. I dealt with Darman back in the Nixon administration, when he was a top aide to Elliot Richardson, one of Nixon's HEW secretaries. Darman is a very bright guy. In fact, it sometimes seems as if he's got an IBM 390 mainframe built up between his ears.

But again, OMB is calling all the shots on health care. President Bush has done a marvelous job on foreign policy, but for most of his first term he hasn't pursued a domestic-policy agenda with much energy. When it comes to health, he basically hasn't been there at all.

Although dealing with a president is sometimes exciting, more often than not you deal with his staff and with the secretaries and assistant secretaries of the departments and agencies. I've known every secretary of HEW and HHS since Elliot Richardson on a first-name basis, and I have felt sorry for every single one of them. Sometimes I've even said to them, "Why did you take this job? And better yet, why do you keep it?"

Take Otis Bowen, Reagan's third secretary of Health and

Human Services, for example. You didn't have to explain anything to Otis—he had practiced medicine all of his life. Incredibly, Bowen was the first physician to serve as secretary since the department was created during the Eisenhower administration.

But Bowen was more than a physician. He had served as a state legislator in Indiana, including several terms as speaker of the Indiana House of Representatives. He later served two terms as Indiana's governor and did quite a job of reforming that state's medical-malpractice laws. After he retired, Reagan asked him to chair the Advisory Council on Social Security, which studied the Social Security, Medicaid, and Medicare programs and made proposals to preserve their financial health and improve their benefit packages. He was appointed secretary of HHS in 1985.

Otis knew the federal government; he understood the legislative process. But most important he was a patient's doctor. Because he had been a practicing physician, a legislator, and a governor, I think Otis Bowen was in a position to do the best job of anybody that's ever been in the job. But the Reagan administration wouldn't let him do it. Here was a man who had the knowledge, the experience, and the motivation to accomplish what doctors and patients in this country want, by God, and his bosses wouldn't let him do it. They treated him abysmally. They had third- and fourth- and fifth-echelon White House staff people reviewing his speeches and telling him what he could and could not say about health care. One day I said to him, "Why in the hell don't you call the president on that private line and tell him to take that damn job and shove it? You have no reason to be that loyal to Ronald Reagan when his people are treating you that way." Otis wouldn't do it, but I wish he had.

Probably the most frustrating secretary I've dealt with was Joe Califano, Carter's first HEW chief. He didn't take orders from anybody, including the president. Philosophically, Califano was very far away from where I was. But we got to be very good friends and still are. Califano used to call me fairly frequently at six o'clock in the morning Chicago time and say, "Jim, I just want to tell you what I'm going to do today, so you won't get caught by surprise."

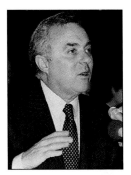

As secretary of Health, Education and Welfare under Carter, Joseph Califano backed an administration plan for national health insurance.

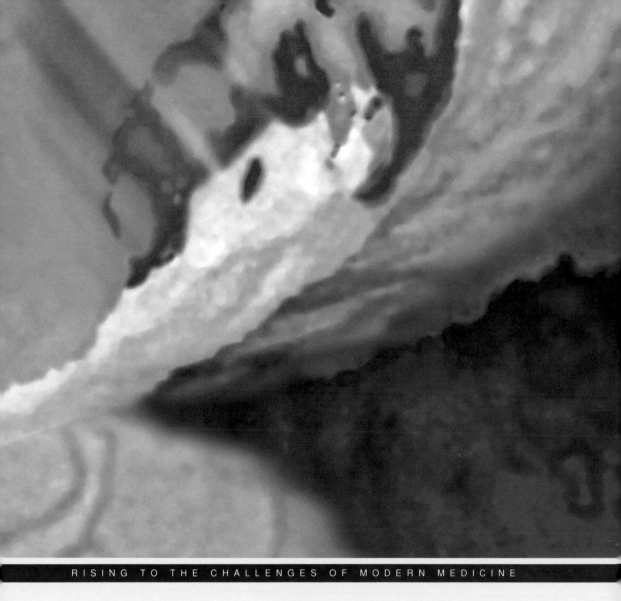

CHALLENGE:

**TO REDEFINE THERAPEUTIC SUCCESS IN MANAGING
THE SYMPTOMS OF CHRONIC ARTHRITIS. SYNTEX RESPONDS...**

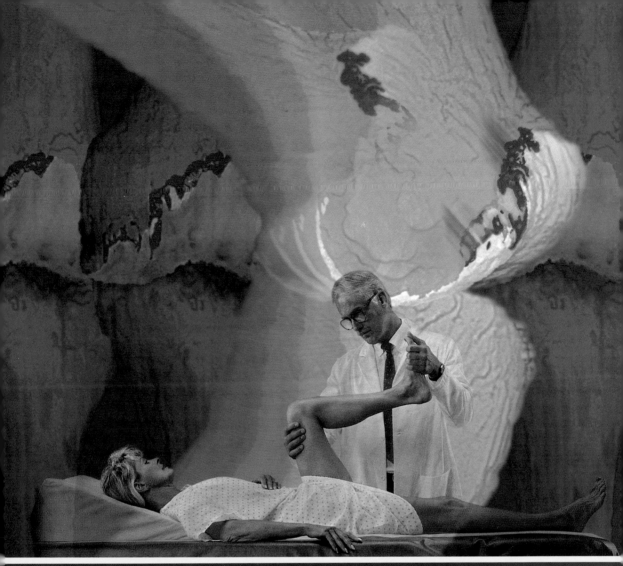

NAPROSYN®
(NAPROXEN) 500 MG TABLETS.

A CONTEMPORARY BENCHMARK OF CHRONIC
ARTHRITIS MANAGEMENT, **NAPROSYN** COMBINES
EFFICACY AND TOLERABILITY FOR THERAPEUTIC SUCCESS.

AS WITH OTHER ANTI-ARTHRITIS AGENTS, THE MOST FREQUENT
COMPLAINTS WITH **NAPROSYN** ARE GASTROINTESTINAL.
SEE "WARNINGS," "PRECAUTIONS," AND "ADVERSE REACTIONS"
SECTIONS OF COMPLETE PRESCRIBING INFORMATION
ON PAGES I-IV OF THE APPENDIX.

SYNTEX

H

Almost without exception I'd say, "Joe, for God's sake, don't do that. Let's talk about it."

Now, I supported a lot of what he did to raise the public's understanding of the dangers of cigarette smoking. For his time, the statements he issued on cigarettes were quite brave. After all, his president was from the South and depended on tobacco-producing states for his electoral base. While Califano was blasting away at cigarettes, the White House political team was flinching and counting the votes going down the drain.

But Califano and I differed when it came to the government's role in health-care delivery. He believed that government regulation was the answer to any problem. He and Carter pushed for a hospital cost-containment bill that would have put the government in charge of setting prices for all hospitals, private and public (thank God that was defeated by Congress). And Califano and Carter pushed for a national-health-insurance bill that would have put the government in charge of insuring all citizens. After what the government did with Medicare and Medicaid, that idea doesn't sound so appealing.

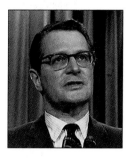

Elliot Richardson served as Richard Nixon's secretary of HEW from 1970 to 1973.

Califano and Carter wound up having a falling-out in 1979, and Joe was fired. That's usually the way it works when you get in a fight with the president.

One of the smartest people I've known was Elliot Richardson, one of Nixon's appointees as HEW secretary. But things were a lot easier in America when Richardson was secretary: the government was expanding, and so was the economy. Richardson only had to worry about figuring out ways to spend all of the money Congress wanted to give him. I think it would be very interesting if Richardson had another shot at being secretary. I have the feeling that he would bring some new and very innovative ideas about health-care financing to the table.

I'm not sure that President Bush's HHS secretary, Louis Sullivan, will fare much better than any of the others did. When it's all cut and dried, Sullivan may find there's a lot of stuff they won't let him do. I'm sure his frustration will be eating him alive.

In real terms, the Bush administration has so far been a continuation of the Reagan years. The government continues to try to regulate the cost of health care without doing a thing about the millions of people who aren't getting enough care. Rather than taking a careful approach to writing good health policy, the government follows what I call the salami method of governing: they slice a little bit here, they slice a little bit there, all to save a few bucks. But when it comes down to it, they don't understand the consequences of all of those cuts. They've created a regulatory system that is so administratively burdensome that many doctors are dropping Medicare patients from their practice.

In many ways, things are getting worse. Policymakers in Washington today—and by that I mean both the president and Congress—are extremely timid. They're all afraid to make any move lest they offend one or more interest groups. As a result they do nothing.

By the middle of Reagan's second term, many members of Congress were tired of always voting to cut programs. There was a pent-up demand for new efforts to help those who weren't getting what they needed. When Otis Bowen joined the Reagan cabinet he wanted to plug the holes in Medicare's acute-care-benefit package and provide protection against the cost of catastrophic illness. This wasn't some theoretical concept for him; he had nursed his first wife through a terminal bout with cancer and had seen how such an illness can drain a family of its life savings.

Bowen convinced the administration to propose a limited catastrophic-insurance bill that would have provided unlimited hospitalization coverage and placed a $2,000 annual cap on the amount of out-of-pocket spending the elderly could incur in any one year. It was a good proposal, but the Democrats in Congress had to put their own mark on the plan; they proceeded to pile on a series of amendments that brought the cost for Part A of the program up to $4.4 billion a year. Many of those amendments were worthwhile—things like prescription-drug coverage, for example. But the government couldn't afford to add $4.4 billion to the annual cost of Medicare, so Reagan and Congress decided to make the elderly pay for the added benefits.

That prompted a huge outcry from senior citizens—particularly those who were rich enough to have to pay the maximum $800 annual premium. It was the worst case of freeloading I had ever seen. A very affluent group of people over 65 killed the catastrophic-health-insurance program for the people who really needed it—300,000 killed the bill for 30 million. It was the damnedest misadventure in democracy that I can think of.

Congress is to blame too. It capitulated when it didn't have to; it knuckled under to a first-class public relations campaign by a minority of the people covered in the Medicare program. But as a result, it's going to be tough for Congress to find the guts to really do what it needs to do to save the program, which is what I'll discuss in chapters 7 and 8.

CHAPTER FOUR

RB-RVS

y the mid-1980s, it had become clear that if organized medicine didn't act soon, the government would keep slicing away at the Medicare budget until there was nothing but table scraps left to finance a system that was already unfair in the way it compensated physicians for the care they provided to Medicare patients. In its rush to enact Medicare back in 1965, Congress had adopted a physician fee system based on historical charges. Fees were set according to what was then "usual, customary, or reasonable." As a result, many of the fee patterns of the mid-1960s—when surgery was the dominant form of treatment and primary care was an underpaid specialty—were still locked in place in the 1980s.

Many of us in organized medicine had argued for some time that there needed to be a redistribution of Medicare revenues among physicians. Simply put, surgeons were being overcompensated for some of the procedures they did and primary-care physicians—internists, GPs, and family physicians—were being undercompensated. The only reason many in medicine were able to live with the inequities in the system was that for a long time, the size of the Medicare pie had been growing each year. But by 1987, the pie had stopped growing.

That fact was brought home by attempts to reduce Medicare fees for what were called "overpriced procedures." In 1988, those geniuses in Washington decided that they would designate certain procedures (things like cataract surgery and transurethral prostatectomies) as overpriced and reduce the fees that were paid. Organized medicine protested—loudly.

It's not that we didn't agree that some fees were too high. It's just that we thought congressmen and federal regulators were the last people in this world who should decide which fees were too high.

So in the early 1980s we began advocating a reexamination of the whole fee structure that had been put in place back in 1965. At first, it was hard to get the attention of Congress, which was preoccupied with budget cutting. But slowly, our allies on Capitol Hill gained ground. By the mid-1980s, Congress was growing tired of the freeze-and-squeeze approach to regulating physicians' fees and was open to the idea of revamping the system. In 1986 it directed the federal Health Care Financing Administration (HCFA) to contract for a study of the relative values of various physician services and devise a new fee schedule based on the resources required for a physician to perform each one. HCFA was to report back in two years.

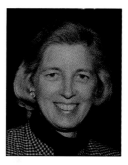

Carolyne K. Davis of the Health Care Financing Administration supervised the awarding of funds to study the RB-RVS.

I favored a move to what came to be called the resource-based relative-value scale, or RB-RVS. There was no doubt in my mind that general practitioners, pediatricians, internists, and many ob/gyns around the country had been methodically and consistently underpaid by insurance carriers and other third-party payers for a very long time.

Surgeons protested, and I didn't blame them—in this kind of ballgame, you get what you can, provided it's honest, fair, and earned. Nevertheless, I thought the nonsurgical groups had been at a disadvantage, and I thought that without RB-RVS or some other kind of relative-value scale, Congress would continue to slice away at payments for the so-called overpriced procedures.

Of course you've got to go back to the 1950s and '60s to realize that although it's got a new title today, the RB-RVS ain't all that new. In the 1960s the California Medical Association developed its own relative-value scale. It was an incredible piece of work. It amazes me even now to think that almost 40 years ago the CMA was able to put together enough people from different specialties for a long enough period of time to formulate that first RVS.

Unfortunately, the Federal Trade Commission got involved and in 1979 stopped everybody from using it. The commission argued that medical societies could not create a payment system that governed their members. It was afraid of the possibility of price collusion, which would violate the federal antitrust statute. But before that happened, Nebraska, New Mexico, and several other states had published their own versions of what was basically the California RVS with new covers. The American College of Radiology, as well as some other specialty societies—pathologists and anesthesiologists, for example—also published their own relative-value scales.

By the mid-1980s organized medicine was ready to give it another try. But this time it was Congress that got things going, with a little push from medicine.

The AMA was interested in helping to conduct the HCFA study. After all, who could be a better judge of the amount of time and work it takes a physician to perform a service? I met with the administrator of HCFA, Carolyne Davis, to talk it over. She said, "Look, the AMA is not going to get this. It's the old fox in the henhouse story. The contract is going to go to some educational institution, but if you want to subcontract, we won't object."

So, when HCFA gave the contract to Harvard economist William Hsiao, we immediately said, "We want to subcontract. We want to be part of this because we believe in it." And to Bill's everlasting credit, he said okay. We helped to bring the specialty societies to the table and ensure that the people they nominated to serve on the panels were the right people to do the job.

The study lasted for nearly three years, and it went very well. Bill would conduct a series of panel meetings with specialists in certain fields—ophthalmology, cardiology, neurology, and the like. They would go down a list of procedures one by one and rate how much time and work went into performing each one. They generally would compare their estimates against the same factors required for a standard procedure—let's say a hernia repair—and indicate whether they thought the procedure took twice as much work, half as much work, or about the same amount of work. There wasn't much professional disagreement about the majority of procedures, though there was a great deal of argument about some of them.

Unfortunately, the American College of Surgeons and

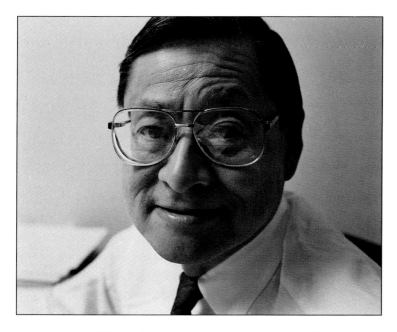

Economist William Hsiao of Harvard won the HCFA contract to formulate the RB-RVS. The new reimbursement system is being imposed in stages, beginning in January 1992.

some of the surgical specialty groups fell off the RB-RVS bandwagon right up front. This came as no surprise to me. Surgeons saw themselves taking a lick no matter how the pie was redivided.

Even if I wasn't surprised, I tell you candidly that when the College of Surgeons pulled out I was upset and disappointed. I thought it wasn't in their best interest to do so. I said to some of their guys, "You're crazy. If you're not going to be at the table when the final document is drawn, don't be surprised if the shaft is bigger."

We had made every effort to make sure the surgeons took part. I talked to Paul Ebert, the executive director of the College of Surgeons, and urged him to participate. Our executive committee met with their executive committee. But the surgeons saw RB-RVS as a real threat to their livelihood. I understood that, but I felt they were simply not acting in the best interest of their members.

Not all of the surgical specialties opposed the RB-RVS. Some, like the thoracic surgeons and the ophthalmologists, felt they weren't getting a fair shake and were able to help because their surgeons were with them. And as it turns out, I think a level of fairness existed despite the fact that not all the surgical societies participated. But I do think the actions of those that didn't set the whole process back.

Other specialty societies—the American Society of Internal Medicine, the American College of Physicians, the Academy of Family Physicians, the American Academy of Pediatrics, and the American College of Obstetricians and Gynecologists—were supportive and really worked at it. That made the RB-RVS fly: they saw the need for it and did the work. The AMA took an umbrella role and coordinated interaction with Hsiao.

There was never any doubt in my mind that some kind of equalization or adjustment would happen because physicians' payments were out of kilter. There's no reason in the world that pediatricians and family docs should be at the bottom of the totem pole. They are the primary point of entry into the health-care system, the primary deliverers of care. They save lives, and they heal people. They see to it that patients get well just as much as the guy who picks up a knife and cuts. My colleague, Jim Todd, who is now executive vice-president of the AMA, liked to say of surgeons, "A chance to cut is a chance to cure." But I would always reply that the chance to make the diagnosis, to write the prescription, to do the follow-up—those, too, are chances to cure.

There were some difficult times along the way to working out the RB-RVS. Every once in a while, just as we'd gotten things quieted down, Bill Hsiao would make a comment to the press or at a meeting, and things would come apart at the seams. The surgeons, for instance, knew going in they were going to take a hit—the big question was what kind of hit it would be. When Bill was quoted as saying the surgeons could lose as much as 60 percent of their Medicare revenues, the surgeons went through the roof, even after Bill disavowed the comments. But eventually things quieted down a bit.

In the end, the final version that went to HHS did not have the kinds of cuts people had feared. The primary-care people didn't get as much as they thought they were going to get, and

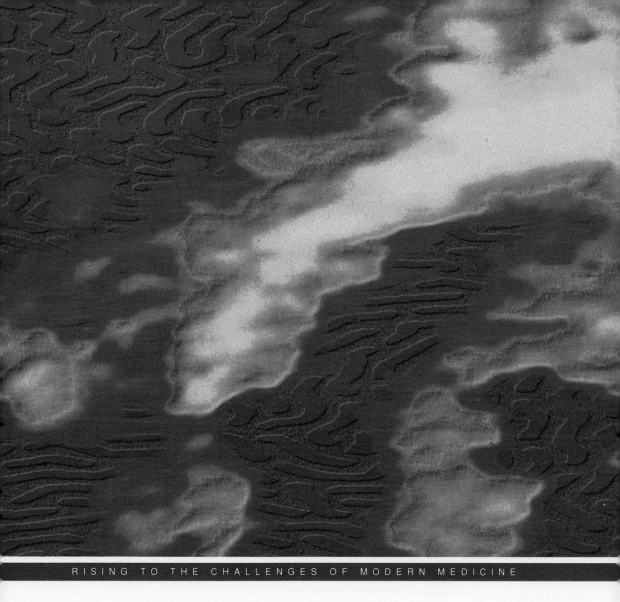

CHALLENGE:

TO ZERO IN ON BOTH CHRONIC STABLE ANGINA AND HYPERTENSION WITH THE NEXT GENERATION OF CALCIUM CHANNEL BLOCKADE. SYNTEX RESPONDS...

🄢 SYNTEX

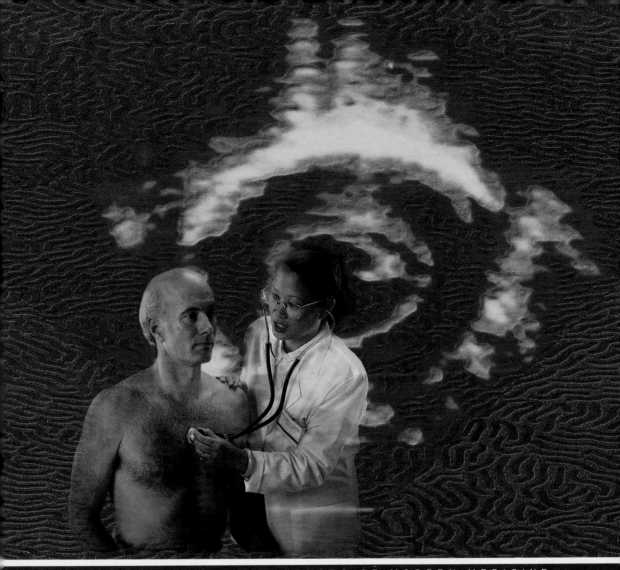

CARDENE®
(NICARDIPINE HYDROCHLORIDE) 20, 30 MG CAPSULES.

A DIHYDROPYRIDINE CALCIUM ENTRY BLOCKER,
CARDENE IS A SOUND CHOICE FOR FIRST-LINE THERAPY
IN BOTH CHRONIC STABLE ANGINA AND HYPERTENSION.

THE MOST FREQUENT ADVERSE EVENTS ARE FLUSHING,
HEADACHE, PEDAL EDEMA, AND DIZZINESS. SEE "WARNINGS,"
"PRECAUTIONS," AND "ADVERSE REACTIONS" SECTIONS
OF COMPLETE PRESCRIBING INFORMATION
ON PAGES XX-XXV OF THE APPENDIX.

the surgeons didn't get cut as much as they thought they were going to get cut. The plan must be pretty good if nobody's fears were fully realized.

But we did get into one last big hassle: the timetable for implementing the RB-RVS. The College of Surgeons was livid not only over the idea that it was going to happen, but that it was going to be put in place in one to three years. They didn't want any part of that; they wanted five years or 10 years. That was unrealistic. Once Congress had made up its mind to do something, it was ludicrous to think they would not insist on implementation within a relatively short time.

But the time-frame question created a hell of a problem anyway in Congress and among the specialty groups. My answer was, "Look, I don't really care if it's one year, two years, or three years. What I care about is we need it. The sooner we get it passed the better, and the sooner we get it implemented the better, because the need is there. We're not going to bleed and die on the floor over whether it's one year, two years, or three years. We just want it done at the most effective rate and one that is attainable." (My concern was that a very short time frame would not be attainable.)

We finally said to Congress, "Three years maximum. If you can do it in less than three years, then let's get on with it." At that point, in 1989, the AMA was saying the same thing that most of the specialty groups, even some of the surgical specialties, were saying. We thought three years was an attainable time frame. The final schedule called for RB-RVS to be introduced over a four-year period, beginning in January 1992.

There had to be an adjustment in the fee schedules; without it we would be faced with an ongoing shortage of people in the primary-care specialties. I believe what I just said and have for a long time, and the best way to do it is with RB-RVS. You have to accept that everybody is not going to be happy. There have to be trade-offs and, on occasion, there have to be decisions made based on gut reaction and emotion. But if you have people who are well-intentioned and who believe that medicine is the sum of its parts, then it can work.

I think that's exactly what happened in formulating the RB-RVS. There were enough people who understood that the pie wasn't going to get much bigger, and that there were great inequities that had been building up over a period of years in the distribution of that pie. And they knew that if you let the government make the necessary adjustments, it would only make a mess.

The RB-RVS study was a classic case of experienced practitioners of medicine involving themselves in the often frustrating process of government policymaking and achieving a better system for themselves, their colleagues, and the future of medicine. There was no way that the paid lobbyists could have achieved the same results, no matter how well they might have made our case.

CHAPTER FIVE

PLAYING HARDBALL

T here are times when you have to throw down the glove and engage in hand-to-hand combat to defend what you know is right and to prevent something that you know is not only wrong but potentially dangerous. You go into such battles knowing full well that you're going to make some people angry. And although you hope that when things cool off you can go back to business as usual, you realize that sometimes that just isn't possible.

In the course of my 16 years at the helm of the AMA, there were many such battles. One sticks out in my mind, maybe because it was one of the last or perhaps because the stakes were so high. Either way, it was a fight that organized medicine decided it must take on despite the risks of angering a new and very popular administration in Washington as well as some of our best friends on Capitol Hill.

In 1989, right in the middle of the RB-RVS negotiations, the Bush administration decided to throw us a curve. In its never-ending hunt for new "savings" to reduce the federal budget deficit, the administration proposed something it called an expenditure target, or ET. The idea, as they saw it, was to impose an annual target for Medicare Part B spending. If actual spending happened to fall beneath that target, everything would be fine. But if spending exceeded the target, the government would take the excess out of the fees paid to physicians the next year.

That's what they said. But physicians knew that ETs (or whatever you wanted to call them) meant one thing—rationing of medical care to our nation's elderly. Under the ET scenario, a physician would have to say at some point to a patient, "Too bad, you didn't make the target."

As with most things in health policy, ETs weren't new. The administration got the idea from the Canadians—yes, those same Canadians the administration criticized for having a system that causes rationing.

The White House had arranged some political cover by getting the supposedly independent Physician Payment Review Commission (PPRC) to come out in favor of ETs. Up until this time, the PPRC had been a very useful group of experts who gave the administration and Congress recommendations on ways to make the Medicare system work better, but the panel hadn't ventured into the political waters of budget cutting. Now, under pressure from the White House, the PPRC put itself right in the middle of one of the biggest fights physicians in this country had ever faced.

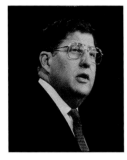

John Sununu, Bush's chief of staff, was furious when the AMA gave his direct telephone number to its members during 1989's expenditure target (ET) fight.

The idea actually came from two guys over in the White House. The first was John Sununu, President Bush's chief of staff. Sununu had been a three-term Republican governor of New Hampshire before Bush asked him to run the White House staff. The AMA hadn't had a lot to do with Sununu when he was in office in New Hampshire, but I had heard about his reputation for being difficult—a reputation he certainly would live up to. The other person behind the ET concept was Bush's director of the Office of Management and Budget, Richard Darman.

Sununu and Darman cooked up the ET idea and decided to spring it on us in July 1989. But they made a serious mistake in their timing. They announced the administration's support for ETs while the AMA's House of Delegates was holding its annual meeting in Chicago. All of the top leaders of the medical profession were in one place along with 400 of the best lobbyists medicine could have—the members of the House of Delegates. These men and women were, and are, committed individuals who know how to make their feelings known and aren't shy about doing so. When Sununu and Darman let it slip that they were supporting ETs, the AMA swung into action.

The first thing we did was print up hundreds of red-and-white lapel buttons saying NO TO ET. Each of the delegates wore one the next day as a sign of solidarity and as a signal to the people watching us that we weren't going to take this one lying down. We then put up big posters around the House of Delegates meeting site urging our members to call Sununu's office and let him know what doctors thought about ETs. And we printed his direct number!

Next, we designed a series of full-page newspaper advertisements that made our point very clearly. One in particular was quite effective: it pictured an elderly woman who looked like she could have been most people's mother or grandmother, with the caption, "Who's going to tell her she's an expenditure target?"

Well, I have to tell you those things really did the trick. For the next three days, Sununu's office was inundated with telephone calls, and so was Darman's. Finally, the two of them called us to the White House for a meeting. With me on our side of the table were Dr. Alan Nelson, the AMA president that year; Wayne Bradley, one of my top vice-presidents; and John Zapp, the head of our lobbying office in Washington. On the other side were Sununu and Darman.

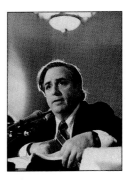

Richard Darman, director of the Office of Management and Budget, played good cop during debates about ETs with AMA officials.

Sununu's blood pressure must have been something like 5,000 over 1,000. He was irate that we had given away his White House telephone number. He looked at me and said, "The next time you're going to do this, tell me first and I'll give you a special telephone number so you don't disrupt my office." Well, we had wanted to disrupt his office. That was the whole point.

In the past at meetings of this type, one of the administration people would usually play good cop and the other one bad cop. This time, Sununu was the bad cop, but he wasn't playing a game; he was mad. I understood why—our ads were working. We had gotten the administration's attention. They had not been listening to our Washington office; they had not been listening to what was coming out of Chicago. The AMA plan was carefully thought out.

We'd been trying to see President Bush for eight months, ever since he'd been inaugurated, and Sununu wouldn't let us in. Now I told Sununu, "You know, this could have

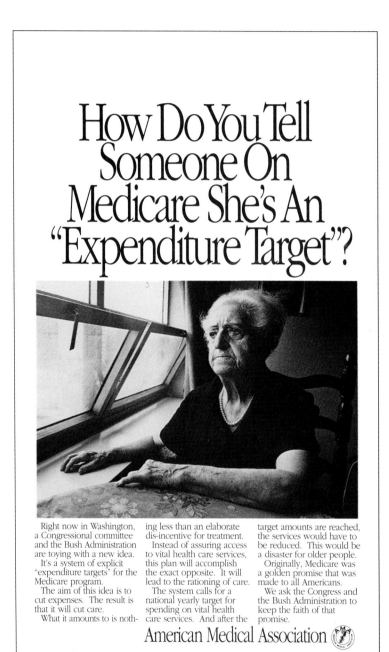

How Do You Tell Someone On Medicare She's An "Expenditure Target"?

Right now in Washington, a Congressional committee and the Bush Administration are toying with a new idea.

It's a system of explicit "expenditure targets" for the Medicare program.

The aim of this idea is to cut expenses. The result is that it will cut care.

What it amounts to is nothing less than an elaborate dis-incentive for treatment.

Instead of assuring access to vital health care services, this plan will accomplish the exact opposite. It will lead to the rationing of care.

The system calls for a national yearly target for spending on vital health care services. And after the target amounts are reached, the services would have to be reduced. This would be a disaster for older people.

Originally, Medicare was a golden promise that was made to all Americans.

We ask the Congress and the Bush Administration to keep the faith of that promise.

American Medical Association

When the White House announced its support for ETs, the AMA retaliated with a series of highly effective newspaper ads to express organized medicine's opposition to the idea.

been avoided if you had just allowed us to go in and see the president."

Well, Sununu got all white in the face, he was so mad, and I shall never forget it. He shouted, "You will never see the president of the United States as long as you make these things political!"

I thought to myself, *Governor, where do you think we came from? The whole damn world is political, and certainly you people are being political.* But I demonstrated the better part of valor and said, "Well, you can solve a lot of these problems if you'll let us see the president."

Meanwhile, Darman was playing the good cop. He kept saying to me, "Jimmy, you're wrong about this. Your numbers are wrong; it's not going to be that bad."

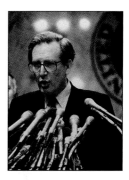

Now I had known Dick Darman as far back as the Nixon administration, when he was a young aide to HEW secretary Elliot Richardson. I'd seen him play this game before; he knew his numbers were phony. I just kept saying, "Listen, Dick, we both know better than that. This is rationing of care. The only way you can make these savings is to reduce the services. That clearly is what you're after, so let's be totally honest about it. We're going to fight it, and we're going to win."

Darman and Sununu were both saying, "No you're not. You're going to lose."

I just said, "We'll see."

Clearly, we weren't getting anywhere at that end of Pennsylvania Avenue. It was time to turn our attention to the legislative branch. We've always had good relations on Capitol Hill—after all, each and every member of Congress has hundreds or thousands of doctors living and practicing back in the district. There on the Hill, our arguments hit home a lot more quickly. There were two fellows in particular we had to deal with in Congress on this ET thing. One was Senator Jay Rockefeller, a Democrat from West Virginia who was chairman of the Senate's Medicare subcommittee. The other was Representative Fortney "Pete" Stark, a California Democrat who chaired the Ways and Means health subcommittee.

Stark is a very odd fellow. He comes from a largely Democratic district in Oakland, California, and made his way to Congress back in 1973 after having owned a bank that featured

Senator John D. "Jay" Rockefeller IV of West Virginia is an outspoken advocate of health-insurance reform.

a big peace symbol on the wall. That attracted all of the hippies and yippies living in Berkeley in those days to put their money in Stark's bank. When he came to Washington, he replaced his hippie clothes with three-piece suits, but he's still an oddball. And Stark's really got it in for doctors. Ever since he was first elected he's taken every opportunity to take potshots at doctors and at the AMA.

Stark immediately got into bed with the administration on the ET proposal. This seemed kind of funny because when he wasn't spewing invective at the AMA, Pete Stark spent a lot of time telling everybody how wrongheaded the Bush administration was on health policy. But on rationing, West and East could agree.

We tried to negotiate with him but he wouldn't talk to me. The word I got was, "The congressman says you're not welcome, and he's not going to talk to you."

I never had the feeling that Pete Stark actually believed what he said. My feeling was that he simply was playing to the media for all he was worth. For some reason, in his mind, being mean and damning physicians, hospitals, and pharmaceutical companies was a great way to sell the public the line that he was protecting consumers' interests.

Our best hope was in the Senate. I set up a meeting with Jay Rockefeller to talk about ETs as well as a PPRC proposal to limit balance-billing charges to Medicare patients. The two issues had become entwined in the budget deal and in Rockefeller's mind. I knew I had my work cut out for me.

When I got in to see him, Rockefeller was not in a good mood. He was distraught that day because his nephew had died in New Mexico, and he was anxious to get to the airport to be with his sister. And he was clearly unhappy about our ad. He was waving it around in my face, saying, "You know, I can buy newspaper ads, too!"

And I said, "Yes, Senator, I know what your name is, and yes, I'm aware that you can buy newspaper ads." In his mind we had stepped on his turf. Again, it was clear that our ads were working. If nobody had paid any attention to them, these lawmakers wouldn't be so unhappy.

Well, Rockefeller calmed down a bit and we had just begun to talk when the buzzer went off signifying there was a vote on

Representative Fortney "Pete" Stark of California is a longtime critic of organized medicine and of physicians. He supported ETs.

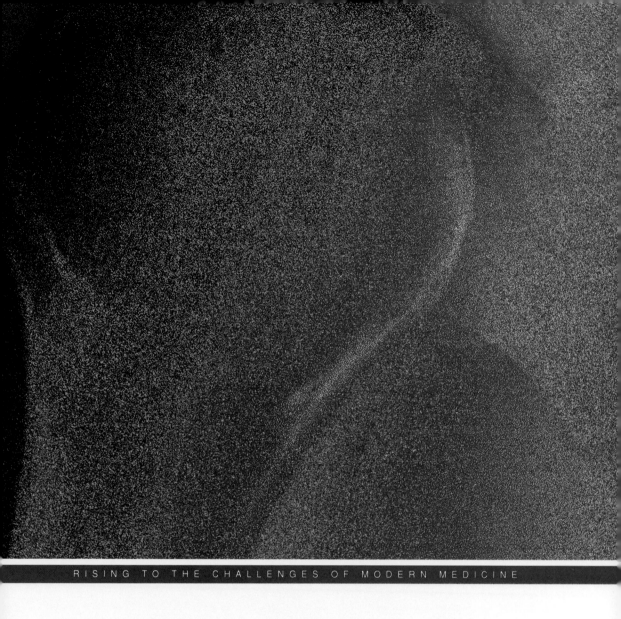

CHALLENGE:

**TO CONCENTRATE ON PROVIDING RAPID RELIEF OF THE SYMPTOMS
OF ACUTE MUSCULOSKELETAL INJURIES. SYNTEX RESPONDS...**

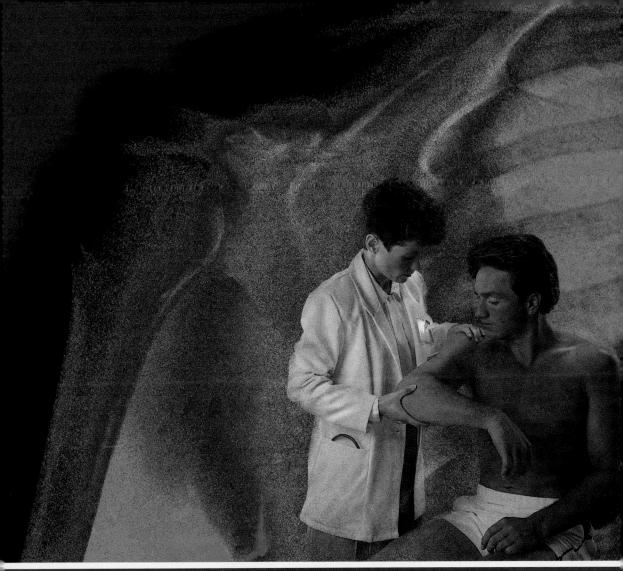

ANAPROX® DS
(NAPROXEN SODIUM) 550 MG TABLETS.

ANAPROX DS WORKS RAPIDLY AND EFFECTIVELY
TO PROVIDE PROMPT RELIEF OF PAIN AND INFLAMMATION DUE TO ACUTE
MUSCULOSKELETAL INJURY — MINIMIZING THE PERIOD OF INCAPACITY AND
FACILITATING A RAPID RETURN TO FULL ACTIVITY.

THE MOST FREQUENT COMPLAINTS ARE GASTROINTESTINAL.
SEE "WARNINGS," "PRECAUTIONS," AND "ADVERSE REACTIONS"
SECTIONS OF COMPLETE PRESCRIBING INFORMATION
ON PAGES IV-VIII OF THE APPENDIX.

the Senate floor. Whenever the Senate is getting ready to vote, a series of buzzers rings in the Senate office buildings to let senators know they have to get over to the floor in the Capitol. Usually these votes are pretty quick, and the senators can either walk over to the Capitol or jump on their underground shuttle to get back and forth quickly. Rockefeller jumped up to go vote, and he told me to come along so that we could finish our talk.

Now, this man is well over six feet tall, and I'm about 5-feet-8 if I'm standing up real straight. Here was this guy taking these great big, loping strides, and I was trying to keep up and talk at the same time.

Finally we got to the shuttle, and it was jam-packed. They were holding the train for Rockefeller, and he told me to climb on, but there was no room. I was thinking, *Climb on where? Do you want me to ride on the front?* I didn't jump on, and off he went.

Rockefeller couldn't continue our discussions that day but we proceeded to meet with his staff and other members of the finance committee over the next few weeks and months. These sorts of negotiations don't occur in one sitting but over a period of weeks. Our staff was meeting with Rockefeller's staff to try to work out a compromise that would save face for both of us. That's the key to any negotiation: both sides have to be able to walk away thinking they've won something.

Meanwhile, we ran our ads again, and wouldn't you know it, the very next day I was supposed to meet with Rockefeller. I got to his office and what was on top of his desk but our ad. He leaned back and said, "I thought you weren't going to do that anymore."

I told him, "Well, I've got a constituency too, and my constituency says these targets are rationing, and I believe it. We're going to keep doing them until we have some sort of agreement on this."

He wasn't quite so mad this time; he understood the constituency problem. Jay Rockefeller is one of the most honorable people that I've ever met. He spent two terms as governor of West Virginia before being elected to the Senate. He doesn't need to be dishonest, and he certainly is not. He clearly is not out to punish doctors. He believes very strongly that patients have got to have doctors. But governing West Virginia also taught him that there is a limit to what you can spend.

As the talks progressed, Rockefeller came around on the rationing argument. He wouldn't support the ET idea as long as we could accept some sort of target for spending. We were able to accept a target as long as it didn't become a cap and as long as the government didn't try to roll back doctors' fees. Rockefeller and I agreed on that, and he promised to include provisions that prohibited any fee rollbacks.

That left only the issue of balance billing. Ever since Medicare was created in 1965, doctors have been able to charge their patients the difference between what the government would pay and their actual costs. Balance billing had been an integral part of Medicare for 25 years, and I was determined to retain it.

The PPRC had devised a plan to limit charges for balance billing. Congress had proposed a limit of 125 percent of the national median, reduced to 115 percent in the second year and 110 percent every year after that. The AMA was dead set against that and told Rockefeller so. But he felt he had given in on ETs and had to have something to walk away with. He was getting impatient; after all we'd been going at this for nearly three months. He leaned across his desk and said, "Well, do we have an agreement?"

I then said, "Wait a minute. All you've been talking about is what's in it for you. But what's in it for my people? You're talking about 115 percent, and that's foolish. It ought to be 135 percent; in fact it ought not be there at all. You should just put the RB-RVS in place and let the patient negotiate. My people have a long history that goes back thousands of years of taking care of people who can't take care of themselves. That's where you ought to be, but that's not where you are. So what's in it for me?"

We haggled and haggled, but finally he said, "A hundred and twenty-five percent."

"That's a mistake," I said, "but I hear you. That's the best you're going to do. Under the circumstances, there's no point in my sitting here and arguing with you. But it's going to come back and bite you because it's wrong."

We wound up taking the 125 percent, but we defeated ETs

despite what Sununu, Darman, and Stark thought. I figured we could always come back and fix the 125 percent later, but once ETs were in place it would have been nearly impossible to fix it. And the AMA did fix the billing limits a year later by getting Congress to raise the floor for primary-care physicians.

So we wound up with a classic political deal. Neither of us could go back to our constituents and say we got everything that we wanted. But neither of us had to go back with our tail between our legs and say we got whipped.

CHAPTER SIX

MEDICAID

or all of Medicare's flaws, at least one good thing can be said for the program: it does pay for health care for senior citizens and the disabled. In other words, it keeps its promises to the people.

The true tragedy of today's American health policy is Medicaid. Designed and enacted at the same time as Medicare, Medicaid was almost an afterthought. Its purpose was supposed to have been to provide government assistance to those who are too poor to pay for their health care or to buy health insurance. Who could argue with that? Not me. I've had many an argument with doctors more conservative than I who say the government has no place paying for medical care. I say, hogwash! If there's anyplace the government should be, it's in the provision of medical care to people who can't afford it—the poor and the near-poor. But Medicaid made that promise without making sure it could be kept.

Lots of mistakes were made in creating Medicaid and in the years since. First of all, no one could decide who should run the thing, so the decision was made by default. By 1963, there were programs in 32 states that helped poor people get medical care, all partially financed by a small federal plan known as Kerr-Mills. But the programs were entirely inadequate, and the poor, who have more health-care problems and need more medical care, had less access to physicians and to hospitals than they did before.

Well, Congress decided it didn't want to take on the issue all by itself. "If the states are already spending some money, let's make sure they keep spending it," some in Congress said. So it set up a program to be run jointly by the federal government and by the states. Each state was allowed to set its own rules on everything from who was eligible to what was covered to how much would be paid to physicians.

When Medicaid started, many of us in organized medicine said, "This is going to be the worst thing anybody has ever seen because the states aren't going to pay the bill." Unfortunately, we were right. The result of Congress's decision is a mishmash of coverage. Some states provide very good coverage: Utah, for example, covers all residents who earn 14.2 percent less than the federal poverty level. Other states are downright miserly: Alabama covers only those who earn 85.4 percent less than the poverty level and provides very few services to those it does cover. Nationally, fewer than half of those who live in poverty [with a yearly income of less than $6,620 for an individual, $8,880 for a family of two, or $13,400 for a family of four] are provided with Medicaid benefits. A 1987 survey says only 13.2 million of 32.5 million Americans living below the poverty line are covered. And yet the program's cost continues to rise—it topped $70 billion in 1990.

To be honest with you, I don't think there is any solution to the Medicaid situation other than getting rid of the program and starting over from ground zero, or federalizing it.

The point of federalization would be to provide some standardization of eligibility, of benefits, and of payment rates. Without that, we will continue to have a program that helps only those who live in states that have a large income base.

My real concerns are access and availability. I am not convinced that Medicaid has made much difference in health care for the poor in spite of all the data that indicate things are better for them today than they were in the past. When it comes to rural America, inner-city America, and parts of the most depressed areas in America, I don't think anybody can honestly demonstrate that things are any better in 1990 than they were in 1960.

One of the things that always has worried me about the Medicaid program is the children. Not only do we not have a uniform eligibility standard, but we have no uniform nationwide program for high-risk pregnancies. On the other hand, statistics show that Medicaid spends a lot of its money on high-risk infants born with life-threatening medical problems. I can

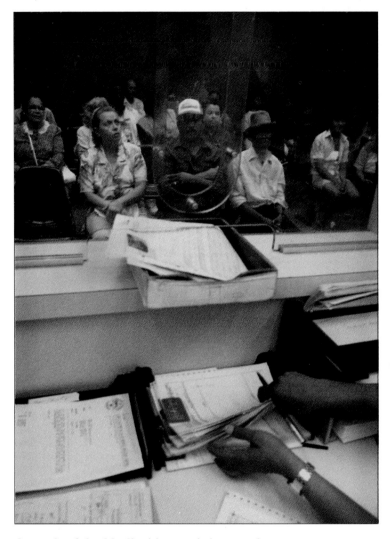

A result of the Medicaid mess is jammed emergency rooms, like this one in New York City, which must handle both critical cases and indigent patients seeking primary care.

argue philosophically within myself that maybe we shouldn't spend all of that money on the high-risk pregnancies because it may be 10, 15, or 20 years before we know whether a child that cost $300,000 to save is going to be even relatively normal. But as a doctor, as a father, and as a grandfather, I can't argue that at all, and I don't make any pretense of trying.

Perhaps in one of those college courses on ethics they can put all the arguments up on a blackboard and decide what to do. But in real life those arguments ain't worth a damn. If you're a doctor and you've got a patient with a problem pregnancy, philosophical arguments fly right out the window.

When you look at all of the promises that were made in 1965—and there were lots of them—and then you stop and look 25 years later, you can see that Medicaid has achieved some positive ends. But at the same time it hasn't come close to achieving what it promised, and without significant reform it won't do so anytime soon.

So that's how I got to the idea of federalization. The first thing to do is standardize eligibility. Today people are eligible for Medicaid if they qualify for Aid to Families with Dependent Children (AFDC) or if they're on Supplemental Security Income (SSI). But states set AFDC standards, and the poor states set them pretty low; only a few of their poor actually qualify for AFDC. That's got to go. I'm not saying we should set eligibility at 100 percent of poverty for all Americans—after all, there are people who can live fairly well at the federal poverty line in areas that don't have the high cost of living that New York or Chicago has. But some sort of standard level of eligibility should be set, and it shouldn't be up to the states to define it.

The next thing that needs to be done is to establish a standard set of benefits. The existing Medicaid program has a general list of benefits that all states must provide, but it lets each state decide how much of each service it will cover. For example, all states have to cover inpatient hospital care. But some states will pay for only 10 days a year. Ten days of hospitalization doesn't cover the needs of a lot of poor people; in those states even the poorest of the poor can't get their medical bills paid by Medicaid. We need a standard benefit package that spells out what is covered and how much of that benefit will be provided.

Finally, we need standardized payment rates for providers of medical care. Some people would say it's pretty self-centered for a physician to expect Medicaid to pay doctors more for caring for Medicaid patients. But face it: in many states payment rates are so low that some doctors simply can't afford to treat a Medicaid patient. At the very least, a program like Medicaid should cover the costs of treating the very poor and provide some margin to cover the cost of running a practice. If we can do that, we can attract some of the best doctors in this country to the program and make sure the poor not only get access to care, but access to the best kind of care that is available.

One way to standardize rates would be to adopt a form of the resource-based relative-value scale. To bring Medicaid provider payment rates up to Medicare standards would require an additional $2.38 billion each year. But for that investment the government could assure that a poor pregnant woman would be able to find an obstetrician/gynecologist who would treat her, provide prenatal care, and deliver her baby.

The end result of Medicaid has been somewhat good, somewhat bad, and somewhat indifferent. But the one constant, it seems to me, is that it's not all good, and it never has been. Medicaid is never going to be all good as long as it's done the way it is now being done and has been done since 1965. Is it salvageable? Yes, absolutely. Is Washington going to salvage it? Hell no, because, politically it's not sexy, and because politicians would have to pay a price.

CHALLENGE:

TO BRING INTO FOCUS THE POWER OF THE FIRST INJECTABLE ANALGESIC NSAID. SYNTEX RESPONDS...

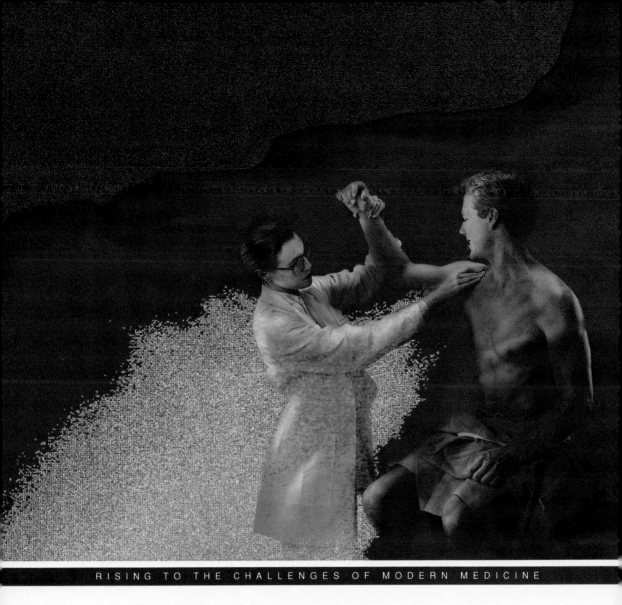

TORADOL® ᴵᴹ

(KETOROLAC TROMETHAMINE) 15, 30, 60 MG.

OUR DEVELOPMENT OF THE FIRST INJECTABLE ANALGESIC NSAID BRINGS
YET ANOTHER BREAKTHROUGH AGENT TO THE SYNTEX THERAPEUTIC LINE.
INDICATED FOR THE SHORT-TERM MANAGEMENT OF PAIN,
TORADOLᴵᴹ PROVIDES NARCOTIC STRENGTH
WITHOUT NARCOTIC COMPLICATIONS.

AS WITH OTHER NONSTEROIDAL DRUGS,
THE MOST FREQUENTLY REPORTED SIDE EFFECTS ARE GASTROINTESTINAL,
WITH SOME GI SYMPTOMS REPORTED BY 3% TO 9% OF PATIENTS
IN CLINICAL TRIALS. SEE "WARNINGS," "PRECAUTIONS," AND "ADVERSE REACTIONS"
SECTIONS OF COMPLETE PRESCRIBING INFORMATION
ON PAGES XVII-XX OF THE APPENDIX.

N

CHAPTER SEVEN

SETTING THE AGENDA

ack in 1982, as budget-cutting fever spread through Washington, I realized that unless medicine offered some realistic suggestions for changes in health-care financing, we would be rolled over by the Reagan Revolution. My idea was to get together a large group of people from organizations representing every conceivable side of the health-policy debate, put them together in one room, and make them work out a proposal for revamping the U.S. health-insurance system that all of them could support and that would stand a chance of getting passed in Congress.

I called this effort the Health Policy Agenda for the American People, and it took five years to achieve a consensus on a plan. I believed then (and still do) that this country needs a health policy to tell us where we are going and how we're going to get there. We had never had a national policy—only bits and pieces of legislation introduced, debated, and sometimes enacted with little thought toward the whole.

This wasn't the first time that the AMA had tried to bring reason to the national health-care debate. In the 1970s we created the National Commission on the Cost of Medical Care, which included people from Congress, labor, management, and medicine. But they only addressed the question of cost and didn't touch on the important issue of access to care.

In the late 1970s, we had the Voluntary Effort, which aimed to control inflation in health-care prices without government intervention. But that, too, was aimed only at the cost side. I was convinced that we needed a true policy, but nobody seemed to be able to put one together. It was certainly clear that the Reagan administration had no interest in establishing a cohesive and coherent policy. It was interested in one thing and one thing only: cost control.

But whenever I talked to physicians about the idea of developing a national policy on health-care access and financing, they immediately went through the roof because they thought we were talking about national health insurance. I finally decided that the AMA was the only group that could bring together the large number of people needed to make it happen. I took the idea to the members of the AMA board of trustees, and they said yes. Then we took it to the House of Delegates, telling them, "We will put this together with a large group of participants, some of whom you don't like. It's going to cost a lot of money and take three or four years." To their everlasting credit, the members of the house approved it without dissent.

The first thing we did was assemble a large steering committee. By the time it was over, there were representatives from some 172 groups of every political stripe involved. We had members from the government, the AFL-CIO, the U.S. Chamber of Commerce, the American Hospital Association, the American Academy of Pediatrics, senior citizens' groups like the American Association of Retired Persons, and consumer groups like the Children's Defense Fund and the Consumer Federation of America. The spectrum of interests was so broad that it was either going to fly early on or it was going to fall apart. People were either going to seriously address the issue or they weren't going to address it at all.

I asked Joe Boyle to chair the whole thing. Joe was then chairman of the AMA board of trustees and would later become executive vice-president of the American Society of Internal Medicine. Joe and I went way back and had fought many a good fight together. I knew he had a sound understanding of the issues and of the political process, and the right temperament to run the show. Joe was, and is, a consensus builder.

After about the second meeting of the steering committee, it became clear to me the members were going to address their mission seriously. They were spending time and money—the AMA had invested a lot of funds in the concept, but the other groups had to spend money too. And they sent good people to the table, people who really made a commitment.

The way Joe Boyle chaired the Health Policy Agenda was magnificent. He allowed no votes in the steering committee; everything had to be by consensus. Sometimes a consensus was hard to come by, and sometimes it took months to get one. And if 172 organizations can come to agreement on a package as comprehensive as the one that eventually emerged, I don't see why the government in Washington can't do the same thing.

So what did the representatives from these 172 groups come up with? First, they designed a basic minimum-benefits package that should be provided to all Americans. Now that may sound easy to do, but let me tell you, it wasn't. Just think about the many special interests involved—one wants mental-health coverage, another wants preventive medicine, another wants respite care, etc. And all of them had good arguments—after all, don't we want all our citizens to have everything they need? But it's become clear that in this country we can't afford to have everything unless we want to spend half of our paychecks just on health care.

Joe Boyle tried to make sure everyone was satisfied, but that proved impossible. People won some things and lost some others. But I think the final product is pretty good. It includes the following:

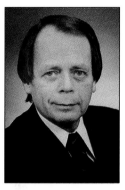

Dr. Joe Boyle, chairman of the AMA's Health Policy Agenda for the American People

Prevention and health promotion

These benefits would include maternal and pediatric care, immunizations, specific medical examinations, and risk-reduction programs.

Acute care

This would provide out-of-hospital diagnostic and therapeutic services, emergency and hospital outpatient services, inpatient hospital services for physical and mental illness, hospice care, short-term care at home or in a nursing home, and rehabilitation facility services.

Chronic care

This provision would furnish long-term health services and extended care in the home or in a nursing home.

We estimated that these benefits could be purchased (in 1988 dollars) for about $110 a month for individuals or $270 a month for a family. We assumed that employers would pick up a percentage of the premium, leaving workers with a manageable monthly expense. The annual deductible expenses would be kept to $200 per individual for hospital expenses and $100 for other services. For families, we suggested a $200 annual deductible for inpatient care and $250 for all other services. Services beyond the annual deductible would be subject to a 20 percent coinsurance charge. To protect against catastrophic-illness expenses, we said there should be an annual limit of $1,500 per individual and $2,500 per family on out-of-pocket expenses.

We did the same thing with dental care. We drew up a basic benefit package that included preventive, diagnostic, and emergency services, routine care, and complex care. Families or individuals could choose how much coverage they needed and add or subtract what they deemed important or unimportant.

Still, there was a lot of complaining about what we didn't include. For example, things like routine physicals, screenings, and exams weren't covered; neither was sterilization. Cosmetic surgery was left out, as were eyeglass and hearing-aid services. There were some tough calls, like leaving out family planning, prescription drugs, and the like. But we tried to limit the benefits package to what is absolutely needed with the understanding that those who could afford more could buy more.

It's easy to pick at what isn't included in the package, but sometimes people lose sight of the achievement there. We were able to design a benefit package that all Americans should have. That's an important contribution to any healthcare debate, and it can help set the stage for action at both the state and national levels.

Our second major proposal was to restructure the Medicaid program so that it serves the people it promises to serve. We wanted to set national standards and national goals. We

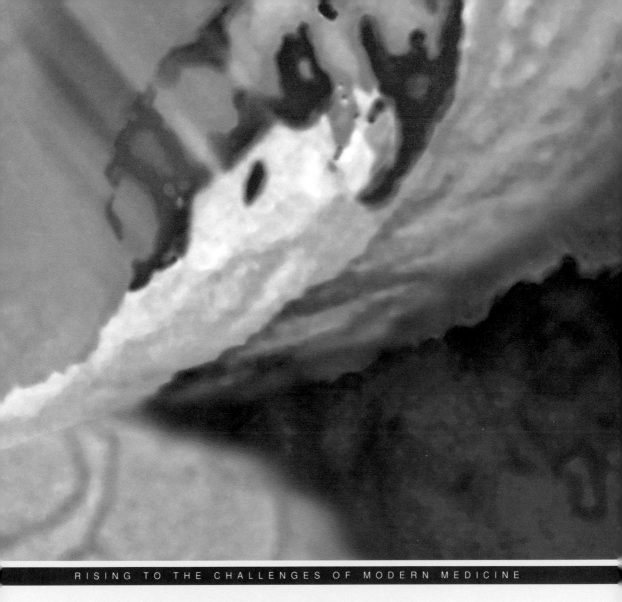

CHALLENGE:

**TO REDEFINE THERAPEUTIC SUCCESS IN MANAGING
THE SYMPTOMS OF CHRONIC ARTHRITIS. SYNTEX RESPONDS…**

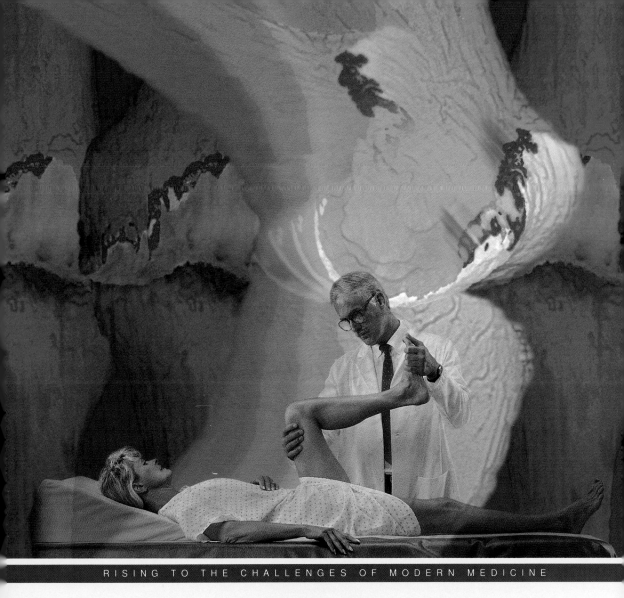

NAPROSYN®
(NAPROXEN) 500 MG TABLETS.

A CONTEMPORARY BENCHMARK OF CHRONIC
ARTHRITIS MANAGEMENT, **NAPROSYN** COMBINES
EFFICACY AND TOLERABILITY FOR THERAPEUTIC SUCCESS.

AS WITH OTHER ANTI-ARTHRITIS AGENTS, THE MOST FREQUENT
COMPLAINTS WITH **NAPROSYN** ARE GASTROINTESTINAL.
SEE "WARNINGS," "PRECAUTIONS," AND "ADVERSE REACTIONS"
SECTIONS OF COMPLETE PRESCRIBING INFORMATION
ON PAGES I-IV OF THE APPENDIX.

SYNTEX

asked Jim Tallon, the majority leader of the New York State Assembly, to chair the ad hoc committee on Medicaid. Jim is one of the most knowledgeable guys I know on Medicaid and a string of other health-care issues. He spent eight years chairing the New York State Assembly's health-care committee and helped to fashion some truly innovative approaches to the health-care problems of the poor. And, as a Democrat, Jim could provide us with the true bipartisan approach we needed to ensure action. After all, we may have had a Republican in the White House, but the Democrats still controlled Congress.

Jim's group recommended eliminating the state-by-state approach to eligibility criteria and replacing it with a national standard, using the federal poverty line as the cutoff point. States would be allowed to provide services to people whose incomes were above the poverty line, but no state could exclude anyone whose income fell below the line. Every state would also be required to adopt what is called a medically needy program to help those who might have sufficient income for ordinary expenses but who would be driven below the national poverty line by large medical bills.

To make sure doctors and other providers participated in the new program, the Tallon group recommended incentives and policies like streamlined paperwork and faster reimbursement to encourage broad participation. It also suggested retaining the long-term-care program, and possibly splitting it off into its own program.

As expected, these kinds of reforms would not come cheap. Jim estimated the cost of revamping Medicaid alone at anywhere from $13 billion to $28 billion a year. The key question was how broad the benefit package would be. Jim set out what I call a smorgasbord approach to the benefits package, offering three options and listing their costs. Option one expands coverage to all those who are uninsured. Option two mandates a standard benefit package for all who are covered. Option three calls for reimbursing providers at market rates. If Congress or some other legislative body didn't like one package, they could choose another. Option one would cost taxpayers about $2.3 billion; option two, between $6.5 billion and $21.5 billion; and option three, $4.4 billion.

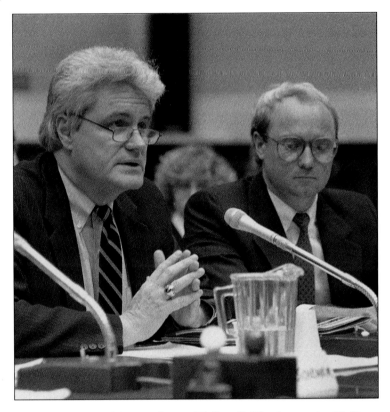

New York assemblyman James Tallon (left), pictured with Kenneth E. Thorpe of the Harvard School of Public Health, chaired the Health Policy Agenda's ad hoc committee on Medicaid.

An expensive but important part of the Tallon report is an attempt to augment provider payments under Medicaid. As he noted, most states pay hospitals, physicians, and other providers under fee schedules set at significant discounts. Such low payments are a frequent cause of limited access to care. Raising Medicaid fees to physicians and hospitals to the level paid by Medicare would cost about $4.4 billion. But as a result there would be an increase of approximately 13.6 million office visits by Medicaid patients, who would then have a doctor to see. That also would ease the load on hospital outpatient departments and emergency rooms, which now see a great number of nonemergency cases.

Now, while Jim was doing his work, another committee was

tackling Medicare. The chairman of this group was former Utah governor Scott Matheson, who unfortunately passed away just last year. Like Jim, Scott was a smart guy who knew health-care issues and knew the political process like the back of his hand. That's why we gave him the difficult job of tackling Medicare reform.

Scott's committee pointed out that the cost of Medicare had skyrocketed well beyond its original estimates. In its first year, Medicare cost $4.6 billion. By 1984, the cost was up to $62.9 billion. (Today, that cost is more than $100 billion.) The annual rate of growth in the program was 8.8 percent in 1987. If things kept going the way they were, the Matheson committee estimated, the Medicare trust fund would be bankrupt by the end of the first decade of the 21st century.

Scott's group made five basic recommendations regarding Medicare:

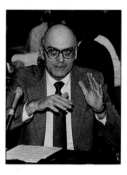

Scott Matheson, governor of Utah from 1977 to 1985, chaired the ad hoc committee on Medicare.

• There should be no further erosion of Medicare benefits.
• Changes in the program should not adversely affect the quality of services.
• Current reserves should be augmented to protect future beneficiaries and the solvency of the trust funds.
• Any increased costs should be borne by all (i.e., the general public, employers, participants, and providers).
• A coordinated approach should contain costs while ensuring access to quality services.

Scott's group very clearly highlighted all of the faults of the Medicare program—the benefits that weren't covered, the cost of care to lower-income senior citizens, and the money that is wasted paying premiums and expenses for people who can well afford to pay for health care on their own.

For example, Medicare now covers the first 60 days a beneficiary spends in the hospital each year. The patient pays for the first day through an annual deductible, and the government pays the full cost of the next 59 days. But once a person exceeds that limit, the patient has to pay one-quarter of the cost for each day through day 90 and one-half of the cost of days 91 through 150. Patients who need more than 150 days of hospitalization in a year have to pay the full freight. That's a terrible burden to place on a person or a family faced with a catastrophic illness.

In his report, Governor Matheson correctly said that if we're going to expand these benefits, we're going to have to change the financing of the program to bring in more money or spend less of it on people who don't need the government's help. In other words, a means test.

There are no dirty words in the phrase *means-test the program.* But in Washington, the term *means test* has taken on a whole different meaning. Knee-jerk politicians immediately charged that we were talking about kicking some folks out of Medicare. But we weren't. What we were talking about was making those who have more money pay more for the care they get. It could be done in many ways, by making them pay a higher deductible or a higher premium. After all, the government now subsidizes 80 percent of Part B premiums for every senior citizen. For many older people that's appropriate—in fact for some, 80 percent isn't enough. But for many others, coverage should be much less or even eliminated. If a 70-year-old retired businessman is earning $150,000 a year on his investments, why should the government subsidize his health insurance? Sure, he paid into the Social Security program while he was working, but that only covers Part A. He should pay the whole cost of Part B, or at least a larger percentage of it.

Scott laid out some other options as well, including raising the payroll tax paid by employers and their workers. That tax now represents about 3 percent of wages; a small increase would produce a large amount of revenue. He also suggested raising excise taxes on such products as cigarettes and alcohol and putting that money into the Medicare trust fund. After all, Medicare ends up spending billions to treat the cancers and other diseases caused by drinking and smoking.

Finally, Scott's group recommended a regular reexamination of all existing regulations "to ensure that they are still needed and that they are consistent with the goals of ensuring access to health-care services." My bet is if they did that, they'd find a lot of these regulations could be wiped off the books without any harm to the government or the patients, and that would do a lot of good for the men and women practicing medicine in this country.

There has been little action on the recommendations of the Health Policy Agenda for the American People. Since the report was issued, Congress and the administration have continued to pursue shortsighted, budget-dominated policies that not only don't improve the system, they make it worse. As long as they're unwilling to take action, then Medicare's going to go to hell. It may take a year, it may take two years, it may take five years, but with the ever-increasing number of the elderly, the shortage of nursing-home beds, and the absence of intermediate-care facilities, it's just a matter of time.

I think the report of the Health Policy Agenda—and in particular the reports by the Tallon and Matheson committees—ought to be required reading for every member of Congress, every staffer in the administration, every science writer in America, every political science course in the United States, and everybody who gives a damn about the legislative aspects of health-care delivery.

One of my greatest disappointments is that it didn't fly. At the time the report was completed in 1987, we were about to start another presidential election campaign, and Congress wasn't ready to debate national reforms.

But one of my great satisfactions is that we were able to complete the report. And as is often the case in Washington, these kinds of reports have a long shelf life and often come back a few years later in a somewhat different form to be the basis for some significant reforms. Today the leaders of Congress and President Bush seem to recognize the need for a national policy and are in the midst of studying the issue. Now, I could tell them not to bother studying any more, just to read the Tallon and Matheson reports. But that wouldn't do any good. They've got to finish their own studies, and when they're done, I wouldn't be surprised if they came to some of the same conclusions. My only hope is that they take action.

CHAPTER EIGHT

A BLUEPRINT FOR CHANGE

I've said before that I'm no believer in saying what's wrong with things without saying what I think should be done about them. I'd be a hypocrite if I ended this book without laying out a series of ideas for what needs to be done to improve the practice of medicine in this country.

I'll tell you right off the bat, however, that none of this comes cheap. Nearly every idea I have will cost us money— either as citizens through higher taxes, or as individuals through more cost sharing in the private sector. I'm no mathematician, but as Jim Tallon and Scott Matheson showed us in their Medicaid and Medicare proposals, the cost of fixing the mess we've got will run into billions of dollars. But let's face it, we're already spending more than 12.2 percent of our country's gross national product on health care, and yet millions of our citizens are getting either no care or barely enough of the care they need. The government, in its attempt to fix things, has only made matters worse. At the same time, it has made it more and more difficult for practicing physicians and other caring professionals to do what they do well—care for patients.

With that somewhat long-winded introduction out of the way, here are some of Jim Sammons' ideas for making the American health-care system better:

Get the private sector to involve itself in solving our access and financing problems.

One of the saddest effects of greater government activity in health-care financing has been the corresponding dramatic decline in the interest and involvement of the private sector: businesses, foundations, charities, and the like. In some ways that's understandable. After all, the government said it would solve our social problems through programs like Lyndon Johnson's Great Society. And we have spent billions of dollars trying to do just that. But sometimes I believe we'd be better off returning to the days when private organizations used their creative abilities to attack such problems.

When I was just beginning to practice medicine in the 1950s I heard about a program begun by the Sears, Roebuck Foundation. After the end of World War II, the demand for quality medical care began to increase beyond the capacity of the system to provide it. So in 1957, Sears set out to increase access to health-care services, particularly in rural areas, by helping small towns build clinics—eventually 163 were established all over the country. The communities were responsible for raising the money to build and equip the clinics and for recruiting the physicians; Sears provided architectural plans and advice on fund-raising.

Because a lot of the clinics wound up being one-man shows, many of the doctors suffered from burnout, and the program eventually failed. I can understand that. You put one doctor in a rural area alone and he or she burns out quickly, with nobody to talk to, nobody to share the patient load with, no easy consultations. But Sears, Roebuck had the right idea in helping to set up these clinics.

The government has been trying for nearly 20 years to solve the same problem. In 1972 it created a program known as the National Health Service Corps and tried handing out scholarships to medical students who promised to practice one or more years in an underserved rural area. But a lot of the students graduated and decided they didn't want to live in some small town when there was so much demand for their services in bigger towns or cities. So they simply defaulted on their obligations.

What's different today? Well, for one thing, there are a lot more physicians out there, and they're still coming out of the schools (about 15,400 are expected to graduate in 1992). But there are fewer opportunities for them because of the concentration of physicians in certain areas. With the economic picture a little hazier, maybe a program like the Sears, Roebuck Foundation's would work better today.

I think you must do everything that you can possibly do in the private sector. When you get to the point where the private sector either cannot or will not solve the problem, it becomes not only an appropriate but a required role of government to step in. But as long as you can do it in the private sector, that's where it ought to be done in the United States of America.

Put more trust in physicians.

For various reasons—most of them involving costs—the past 20 years have witnessed the development of a corps of professional doctor watchers, people whose job it is to look over the shoulders of physicians and other health-care professionals to make sure they're not doing too much or too little. Many of these efforts are well-intentioned, but they have succeeded only in putting a series of barriers between doctors and their patients. We've got peer review organizations, mandatory second opinions, preadmission screening, postdischarge review—you name it.

Have any of these efforts improved the overall quality of medical care? No, they haven't. Can today's system of peer review be improved? No, it cannot. Should it be eliminated? Yes, it should.

Don't get me wrong; I'm not saying we don't need a little oversight. After all, there are some bad apples out there. The problem is, the government and some of these insurance companies act as if the whole barrel is rotten, and they treat every doctor like a worm.

Take a look at the growth in managed care, for instance. Today nearly one-quarter of the American public gets its health care from an HMO or a PPO or some other form of managed care. I have a lot of problems with managed care both as a doctor and as a patient. My problem isn't with the concept. My

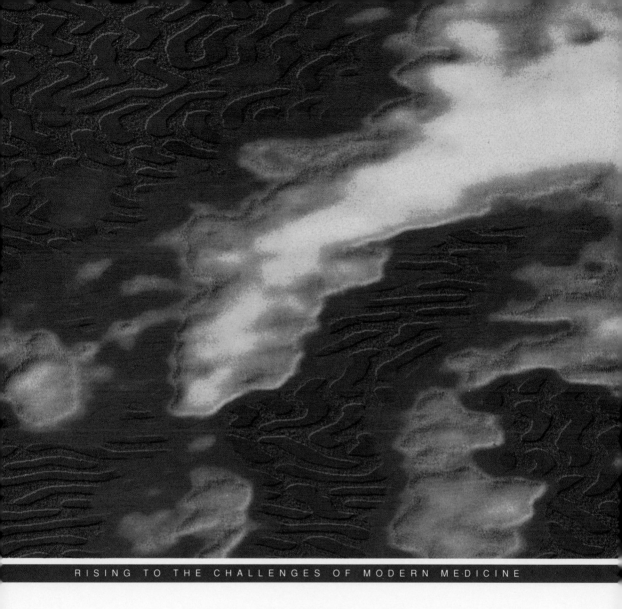

CHALLENGE:

**TO ZERO IN ON BOTH CHRONIC STABLE ANGINA
AND HYPERTENSION WITH THE NEXT GENERATION OF CALCIUM
CHANNEL BLOCKADE. SYNTEX RESPONDS...**

SYNTEX

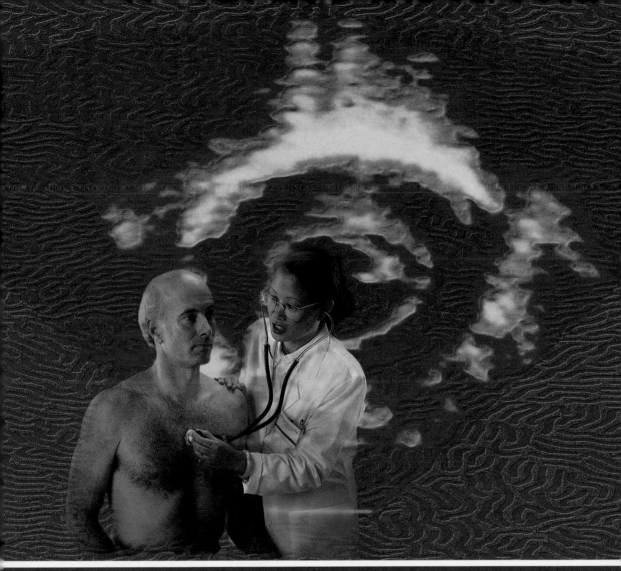

CARDENE®
(NICARDIPINE HYDROCHLORIDE) 20, 30 MG CAPSULES.

A DIHYDROPYRIDINE CALCIUM ENTRY BLOCKER,
CARDENE IS A SOUND CHOICE FOR FIRST-LINE THERAPY
IN BOTH CHRONIC STABLE ANGINA AND HYPERTENSION.

THE MOST FREQUENT ADVERSE EVENTS ARE FLUSHING,
HEADACHE, PEDAL EDEMA, AND DIZZINESS. SEE "WARNINGS,"
"PRECAUTIONS," AND "ADVERSE REACTIONS" SECTIONS
OF COMPLETE PRESCRIBING INFORMATION
ON PAGES XX-XXV OF THE APPENDIX.

SYNTEX

R

problem is with the use of preadmission certification and the interposition of a third party between the doctor and the patient—a third party who has not seen the patient, has not examined the patient, and does not have all of the knowledge about the patient that the doctor has. That just drives me up the wall.

There have been a lot of misconceptions about medicine's views on HMOs and other forms of managed care. As the field was developing in the late '60s and early '70s, many people accused the AMA and state medical societies of trying to prevent the development of HMOs. Nothing could be further from the truth. My father was a railroad man, working for the Central Georgia Railroad, and when I was a little kid, the railroad had a hospital in Savannah and railroad doctors in every town in which there was a depot.

What the AMA fought so vigorously to eliminate in the early '70s was the use of federal funds to create a single form of HMO. We did not believe that federal funds should be used to push one form of practice above all others. But the government was insisting that all HMOs be created alike. I would have felt the same way if federal money was being spent to build private, individual practices. I don't think that's appropriate. We fought that and lost, and a lot of federal money was spent on sponsoring HMOs.

Do something about long-term care.

Take a look at the demographic studies. They all show the same thing: American society is aging, and aging quickly. The fastest-growing group among the elderly today is composed of people over the age of 85; the slowest-growing group in society as a whole is people aged 5 to 24. In 1980, about 11 percent of the population was over age 64; by the year 2020, that will be up to 18 percent. And when the youngest baby boomers reach retirement age in 2030, one of five Americans will be over the age of 64.

What does this mean? Well, of course it means there will be a greater demand for health care. Senior citizens have always required more care and they always will, despite improved lifestyles and the like. But the type of care they will need will be different from the type of care they get today. There will be a much greater demand for home-care services by elderly people who don't want to end up in nursing homes (although there will still be a need for nursing homes and other forms of long-term care).

As a nation, we aren't ready for this change. Although most Americans have good insurance coverage for acute illness, there is very little coverage for long-term care. I've long been a proponent of the greater use of private insurance to cover such costs. But today, less than 2 percent of bills for extended care are paid by private insurers. Instead, Medicaid, a program that was designed for the young and poor, has become a long-term-care program for the poor, the near-poor, and even the middle class.

Thank God we've got some insurance companies that bit the bullet and said, "We're going to try long-term-care policies." I argued and fought and insisted that the insurance carrier for the AMA develop this type of program for the members. It took two and a half years to get it done, and the company's actuaries were just chewing their fingernails. But as a result, the AMA has one of the best long-term-care insurance programs that I've ever seen. Unfortunately it's not replicated in the general population.

But long-term care is needed by the young and the middle-aged as well as the elderly. That was my concept a few years ago when I insisted that the AMA obtain long-term-care coverage for its members. I said, "You're not going to limit it to the seniors. Doctors of all ages and their wives and their children fall out of trees, get in car wrecks." We haven't yet gotten it to the children, but I was told the other day it looks like we might get there soon. We've got to stop addressing some of these problems on a demographic basis that has no legitimacy.

Revise the Medicaid system.

As Jim Tallon so accurately pointed out, the existing Medicaid program neither serves the people it was designed to serve nor provides practitioners of medicine with any incentive to participate. Years of fiddling around the margins have brought us no closer to a fully operating program for the poor. What is needed is an overhaul. Politicians hate to admit they've done something wrong, but there are few members of Congress today who could argue that Medicaid is working well. There certainly aren't many governors who would make that argument.

National standards for eligibility, benefits, and provider payments must be created. Using the federal poverty line for the majority of Americans is a good place to start, but we also must take care of those with higher incomes but catastrophic medical bills. Provider payments should be patterned after the resource-based relative-value scale recently adopted by Medicare. It is a system that has the support of the professions and has been shown to accurately reflect the work that goes into treatment.

Federal legislators and the president must be willing to admit that any Medicaid reform will cost more money. Americans will accept higher taxes if they are assured that the money is going for health care. I don't know many people who would object to paying a few dollars more each year so that poor women, children, and others could receive a minimum level of medical care.

Use a true financial-capability test for Medicare.

It's time to stop the freeloading. Medicare was created to help elderly Americans pay their medical bills at a time when a great majority of those over age 65 were unable to pay for any care. Today, more than 25 years later, the majority of our senior citizens are quite capable of meeting their medical costs. In fact, people over 50 control half of all discretionary income in this country, and 77 percent of all financial assets. What most of them really need is a form of catastrophic-illness coverage so they don't have to worry about wiping out their entire savings when a serious illness strikes.

By reducing the government's subsidy for those earning over a certain income each year, we could spend more of the Medicare budget on those who most need its help. This also would alleviate some of the burden on the Medicaid program, which now picks up the Medicare premium and deductible charges for several million elderly individuals who are below the poverty line. That money would be better spent on the poor young women and children for whom Medicaid was designed.

The extra money could also be used to plug the serious holes in Medicare's benefit package. Congress could restore the catastrophic-insurance benefits it wrongly repealed in 1989 and add other important benefits that seniors now must purchase on their own—things like outpatient prescription drugs, hearing aids, and the like.

Stabilize the federal role in graduate medical education.

A decade of salami-slicing has left the medical education community in disarray. When the 1980s began, most of our major medical schools and teaching hospitals could rely on the government as a stable source of funding to help them train our next generation of physicians and other health professionals. Today that can't be said. In the name of deficit reduction, the government has been shunning its responsibility to help educate doctors. Before the situation deteriorates any further, an understanding must be reached that the government will honor its commitment to medical education.

Stabilize the funding of biomedical research.

The 1980s were a decade of frustration for biomedical researchers. After nearly 40 years of progressive growth in government support for research through the National Institutes of Health and the Alcohol, Drug Abuse, and Mental Health Administration, Washington began to retreat on its vital obligations to subsidize the research community. As a result, many deserving researchers are struggling to find funding for their work.

A lack of foresight by those in elected and appointed office should not condemn our future generations to illness and death. Money spent today for medical research produces great improvements in life expectancy and the quality of life of our citizens and people around the globe.

A particularly important element of stabilizing biomedical research is the restoration of decision-making authority to the medical experts at NIH and other research agencies. That authority was taken away during the Reagan administration and put in the hands of political budget crunchers. As a result, there has been a loss of control by those who know research best—the scientists. The director of the NIH must be able to control her budget and make the decisions necessary to continue our remarkable progress against disease and disability.

Reinstitute the notion of individual responsibility.

With the government's emphasis on paying for medical care to treat illness, there has been a concomitant loss of emphasis on actions individuals can take to improve their own health. The idea of preventive medicine gets a lot of lip service in Washington, but when push comes to shove, there is little real support. Medical research has shown that changes in individual behavior can make a tremendous difference in the health of the individual and of the population. Just look at the progress we've made against such illnesses as lung cancer. Was that progress the result of improvements in the treatment of cancer? To some degree, yes. But more important has been the change in Americans' behavior, the reduction in smoking that has occurred over these last 30 years.

The medical profession must continue to push for greater individual responsibility, and our government must assist by putting federal dollars behind the effort.

Rapidly implement the resource-based relative-value scale.

We fought hard to gain enactment of the landmark reform of Medicare's physician-payment system in 1989. Two years later we still are waiting for the system to be put in place. Under the terms of the law, the RB-RVS goes into effect on January 1, 1992, and will continue to be phased in through 1996. That schedule must be met if the physicians of this country are to have any faith in the word of their government. And the RB-RVS must be continually improved. We must not sit back on our heels and allow this system to become as obsolete as the customary-prevailing-reasonable system it replaced.

Make sure the money we spend is spent well.

There have been a lot of wrongheaded attempts at controlling the cost of medical care by simply paying less for the care that we deliver. That has not helped curb the cost of care; it has simply caused health-care providers to shift the costs of participating in federal programs onto private payers and has made the practice of medicine more difficult.

It is time, therefore, to examine ways to control costs while improving the care provided to our citizens. And medicine must lead the way.

We have begun a process to evaluate the effectiveness of the methods we use to treat illnesses to see if they are the best methods. This will eventually lead to the creation of practice parameters for the hundreds of thousands of working doctors in this country.

Now, my greatest concern about this process, which was begun by the profession, is that government will use the results of our work as a justification for slashing away at its own spending. That is not the purpose of practice parameters, and any such attempt would torpedo the whole process. It may be true that our work will show that some expensive procedures are not as effective as other, less expensive ones. But at the same time, we may well find that certain less expensive methods are not as effective as more costly procedures. If we let our efforts be guided by dollar signs, the only result will be disaster.

Create a national commitment to "we, the people" to take care of those who are truly not able to care for themselves.

If the 1980s taught us anything, it is that we as Americans cannot care only about ourselves. That decade of greed is over, and it is time to return to a sense of community and family. I believe the American public is willing to help those who need help. It is time for elected and appointed officials to realize that it is not political suicide to ask more of our people and to tell them, yes, it will cost more money but that money will be well spent.

Create a national panel—appointed by the president—to answer the following questions:

When we buy health care, what exactly are we buying?
Do we know the true cost of what we are buying?
Is it what we need?
Is it worth the price?
Are we willing to let the private sector do it?
Who pays?
How?

Each of us will have our list of what we as individuals would do. My list, like yours, changes from time to time as we address one or another area of the system. The opportunity we have is to help guide and implement those changes that are necessary, desirable, and obtainable. Failing this, we will have learned nothing from history.

Additional Copies

To order copies of *Inside Medical Washington* for friends or colleagues, please write to The Grand Rounds Press, Whittle Books, 333 Main Ave., Knoxville, Tenn. 37902. Please include the recipient's name, mailing address, and, where applicable, primary specialty and ME number.

For a single copy, please enclose a check for $21.95 plus $1.50 for postage and handling, payable to The Grand Rounds Press. When ordering 10 or more books, enclose $20.95 for each plus $5 for postage and handling; for orders of 50 or more books, enclose $19.95 for each plus $20 for postage and handling. For more information about The Grand Rounds Press, please call 800-765-5889.

Also available, at the same prices, are copies of the previous books from The Grand Rounds Press:
The Doctor Watchers by Spencer Vibbert
The New Genetics by Leon Jaroff
Surgeon Koop by Gregg Easterbrook

Please allow four weeks for delivery.
Tennessee residents must add 7¾ percent sales tax.

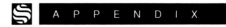

NAPROSYN® (naproxen)

Tablets and Suspension

DESCRIPTION

NAPROSYN® (naproxen) tablets for oral administration each contain 250 mg, 375 mg or 500 mg of naproxen. NAPROSYN suspension for oral administration contains 125 mg/5 mL of naproxen. NAPROSYN is a member of the arylacetic acid group of nonsteroidal anti-inflammatory drugs.

The chemical name for naproxen is 2-naphthaleneacetic acid, 6-methoxy-α-methyl-(+)-

It has the following structure:

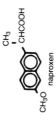

naproxen

Naproxen is an odorless, white to off-white crystalline substance. It is lipid soluble, practically insoluble in water at low pH and freely soluble in water at high pH.

Each tablet contains naproxen, the active ingredient, with the following inactive ingredients: croscarmellose sodium, iron oxides, magnesium stearate and povidone.

NAPROSYN suspension for oral administration contains 125 mg/5 mL of naproxen, the active ingredient, in a vehicle of FD&C Yellow #6, fumaric acid, imitation orange flavor, imitation pineapple flavor, magnesium aluminum silicate, methylparaben, purified water, sodium chloride, sorbitol solution and sucrose.

CLINICAL PHARMACOLOGY

NAPROSYN (naproxen) is a nonsteroidal anti-inflammatory drug with analgesic and antipyretic properties. Naproxen sodium, the sodium salt of naproxen, has been developed as an analgesic because it is more rapidly absorbed. The naproxen anion inhibits prostaglandin synthesis but beyond this its mode of action is unknown.

Naproxen is rapidly and completely absorbed from the gastrointestinal tract. After administration of naproxen, peak plasma levels of naproxen anion are attained in 2 to 4 hours, with steady-state conditions normally achieved after 4-5 doses. The mean biological half-life of the anion in humans is approximately 13 hours, and at therapeutic levels it is greater than 99% albumin bound. At doses of naproxen greater than 500 mg/day there is a lack of dose proportionality due to an increase in clearance caused by saturation of proteins at higher doses. Approximately 95% of the dose is excreted in the urine, primarily as naproxen, 6-0-desmethyl naproxen or their conjugates. The rate of excretion has been found to coincide closely with the rate of drug disappearance from the plasma. The drug does not induce metabolizing enzymes.

In children of 5 to 16 years of age with arthritis, plasma naproxen levels following a 5 mg/kg single dose of suspension were found to be similar to those found in normal adults following a 500 mg dose. The terminal half-life appears to be similar in children and adults. Pharmacokinetic studies of naproxen were not performed in children of less than 5 years of age.

The drug was studied in patients with rheumatoid arthritis, osteoarthritis, juvenile arthritis, ankylosing spondylitis, tendinitis and bursitis, and acute gout. It is not a corticosteroid. Improvement in patients treated for rheumatoid arthritis has been demonstrated by a reduction in joint swelling, a reduction in pain, a reduction in duration of morning stiffness, a reduction in disease activity as assessed by both the investigator and patient, and by increased mobility as demonstrated by a reduction in walking time.

analgesic drugs induce the syndrome of asthma, rhinitis, and nasal polyps. Both types of reactions have the potential of being fatal. Anaphylactoid reactions to NAPROSYN, ANAPROX or ANAPROX DS, whether of the true allergic type or the pharmacologic idiosyncratic (e.g., aspirin syndrome) type, usually but not always occur in patients with a known history of such reactions. Therefore, careful questioning of patients for such things as asthma, nasal polyps, urticaria, and hypotension associated with nonsteroidal anti-inflammatory drugs before starting therapy is important. In addition, if such symptoms occur during therapy, treatment should be discontinued.

WARNINGS

Risk of GI Ulceration, Bleeding and Perforation with NSAID Therapy:

Serious gastrointestinal toxicity such as bleeding, ulceration, and perforation, can occur at any time, with or without warning symptoms, in patients treated chronically with NSAID therapy. Although minor upper gastrointestinal problems, such as dyspepsia, are common, usually developing early in therapy, physicians should remain alert for ulceration and bleeding in patients treated chronically with NSAIDs even in the absence of previous GI tract symptoms. In patients observed in clinical trials of several months to two years duration, symptomatic upper GI ulcers, gross bleeding or perforation appear to occur in approximately 1% of patients treated for 3-6 months, and in about 2-4% of patients treated for one year. Physicians should inform patients about the signs and/or symptoms of serious GI toxicity and what steps to take if they occur.

Studies to date have not identified any subset of patients not at risk of developing peptic ulceration and bleeding. Except for a prior history of serious GI events and other risk factors known to be associated with peptic ulcer disease, such as alcoholism, smoking, etc., no risk factors (e.g., age, sex) have been associated with increased risk. Elderly or debilitated patients seem to tolerate ulceration or bleeding less well than other individuals and most spontaneous reports of fatal GI events are in this population. Studies to date are inconclusive concerning the relative risk of various NSAIDs in causing such reactions. High doses of any NSAID probably carry a greater risk of these reactions, although controlled clinical trials showing this do not exist in most cases. In considering the use of relatively large doses (within the recommended dosage range), sufficient benefit should be anticipated to offset the potential increased risk of GI toxicity.

PRECAUTIONS

General:

NAPROSYN (NAPROXEN) SHOULD NOT BE USED CONCOMITANTLY WITH THE RELATED DRUG ANAPROX OR ANAPROX DS (NAPROXEN SODIUM) SINCE THEY BOTH CIRCULATE IN PLASMA AS THE NAPROXEN ANION.

Renal Effects: As with other nonsteroidal anti-inflammatory drugs, long-term administration of naproxen to animals has resulted in renal papillary necrosis and other abnormal renal pathology. In humans, there have been reports of acute interstitial nephritis with hematuria, proteinuria, and occasionally nephrotic syndrome.

A second form of renal toxicity has been seen in patients with prerenal conditions leading to a reduction in renal blood flow or blood volume, where the renal prostaglandins have a supportive role in the maintenance of renal perfusion. In these patients, administration of a nonsteroidal anti-inflammatory drug may cause a dose-dependent reduction in prostaglandin formation and may precipitate overt renal decompensation. Patients at greatest risk of this reaction are those with impaired renal function, heart failure, liver dysfunction, those taking diuretics, and the elderly. Discontinuation of nonsteroidal anti-inflammatory therapy is typically followed by recovery to the pretreatment state.

NAPROSYN and its metabolites are eliminated primarily by the kidneys, therefore, the drug should be used with great caution in patients with significantly impaired renal function and the monitoring of serum creatinine and/or creatinine clearance is advised in these patients. Caution should be used if the drug is given to patients with creatinine clearance of less than 20 mL/minute because accumulation of naproxen metabolites has been seen in such patients.

Chronic alcoholic liver disease and probably other forms of cirrhosis reduce the total plasma concentration of naproxen, but the plasma concentration of unbound naproxen

In patients with osteoarthritis, the therapeutic action of the drug has been shown by a reduction in joint pain or tenderness, an increase in range of motion in knee joints, increased mobility as demonstrated by a reduction in walking time, and improvement in capacity to perform activities of daily living impaired by the disease.

In clinical studies in patients with rheumatoid arthritis, osteoarthritis, and juvenile arthritis, the drug has been shown to be comparable to aspirin and indomethacin in controlling the aforementioned measures of disease activity, but the frequency and severity of the milder gastrointestinal adverse effects (nausea, dyspepsia, heartburn) and nervous system adverse effects (tinnitus, dizziness, lightheadedness) were less than in both the aspirin- and indomethacin-treated patients. It is not known whether the drug causes less peptic ulceration than aspirin.

In patients with ankylosing spondylitis, the drug has been shown to decrease night pain, morning stiffness and pain at rest. In double-blind studies the drug was shown to be as effective as aspirin, but with fewer side effects.

In patients with acute gout, a favorable response to the drug was shown by significant clearing of inflammatory changes (e.g., decrease in swelling, heat) within 24-48 hours, as well as by relief of pain and tenderness.

The drug may be used safely in combination with gold salts and/or corticosteroids; however, in controlled clinical trials, when added to the regimen of patients receiving corticosteroids it did not appear to cause greater improvement over that seen with corticosteroids alone. Whether the drug could be used in conjunction with partially effective doses of corticosteroid for a "steroid-sparing" effect has not been adequately studied. When added to the regimen of patients receiving gold salts the drug did result in greater improvement. Its use in combination with salicylates is not recommended because data are inadequate to demonstrate that the drug produces greater improvement over that achieved with aspirin alone. Further, there is some evidence that aspirin increases the rate of excretion of the drug.

Generally, improvement due to the drug has not been found to be dependent on age, sex, severity or duration of disease.

In clinical trials in patients with osteoarthritis and rheumatoid arthritis comparing treatments of 750 mg per day with 1,500 mg per day, there were trends toward increased efficacy with the higher dose and a more clearcut increase in adverse reactions, particularly gastrointestinal reactions severe enough to cause the patient to leave the trial, which approximately doubled.

The drug was studied in patients with mild to moderate pain, and pain relief was obtained within 1 hour. It is not a narcotic and is not a CNS-acting drug. Controlled double-blind studies have demonstrated the analgesic properties of the drug in, for example, post-operative, post-partum, orthopedic and uterine contraction pain and dysmenorrhea. In dysmenorrheic patients, the drug reduces the level of prostaglandins in the uterus, which correlates with a reduction in the frequency and severity of uterine contractions. Analgesic action has been shown by such measures as a reduction of pain intensity scores, increase in pain relief scores, decrease in numbers of patients requiring additional analgesic medication, and delay in time for required remedication. The analgesic effect has been found to last for up to 7 hours.

In ^{51}Cr blood loss and gastroscopy studies with normal volunteers, daily administration of 1,000 mg of the drug has been demonstrated to cause statistically significantly less gastric bleeding and erosion than 3,250 mg of aspirin.

INDICATIONS AND USAGE

NAPROSYN (naproxen) is indicated for the treatment of rheumatoid arthritis, osteoarthritis, juvenile arthritis, ankylosing spondylitis, tendinitis and bursitis, and acute gout. It is also indicated in the relief of mild to moderate pain, and for the treatment of primary dysmenorrhea.

CONTRAINDICATIONS

The drug is contraindicated in patients who have had allergic reactions to NAPROSYN® (naproxen), ANAPROX® (naproxen sodium) or ANAPROX® DS (naproxen sodium). It is also contraindicated in patients in whom aspirin or other nonsteroidal anti-inflammatory/

is increased. Caution is advised when high doses are required and some adjustment of dosage may be required in these patients. It is prudent to use the lowest effective dose. Studies indicate that, although total plasma concentration of naproxen is unchanged, the unbound plasma fraction of naproxen is increased in the elderly. Caution is advised when high doses are required and some adjustment of dosage may be required in elderly patients. As with other drugs used in the elderly, it is prudent to use the lowest effective dose.

As with other nonsteroidal anti-inflammatory drugs, borderline elevations of one or more liver tests may occur in up to 15% of patients. These abnormalities may progress, may remain essentially unchanged, or may be transient with continued therapy. The SGPT (ALT) test is probably the most sensitive indicator of liver dysfunction. Meaningful (3 times the upper limit of normal) elevations of SGPT or SGOT (AST) occurred in controlled clinical trials in less than 1% of patients. A patient with symptoms and/or signs suggesting liver dysfunction, or in whom an abnormal liver test has occurred, should be evaluated for evidence of the development of more severe hepatic reaction while on therapy with this drug. Severe hepatic reactions, including jaundice and cases of fatal hepatitis, have been reported with this drug as with other nonsteroidal anti-inflammatory drugs. Although such reactions are rare, if abnormal liver tests persist or worsen, if clinical signs and symptoms consistent with liver disease develop, or if systemic manifestations occur (e.g., eosinophilia, rash, etc.), this drug should be discontinued.

If the steroid dosage is reduced or eliminated during therapy, the steroid dosage should be reduced slowly and the patients must be observed closely for any evidence of adverse effects, including adrenal insufficiency and exacerbation of symptoms of arthritis.

Patients with initial hemoglobin values of 10 grams or less who are to receive long-term therapy should have hemoglobin values determined periodically.

Peripheral edema has been observed in some patients. For this reason, the drug should be used with caution in patients with fluid retention, hypertension or heart failure.

NAPROSYN suspension contains 8 mg/mL of sodium. This should be considered in patients whose overall intake of sodium must be restricted.

The antipyretic and anti-inflammatory activities of the drug may reduce fever and inflammation, thus diminishing their utility as diagnostic signs in detecting complications of presumed non-infectious, non-inflammatory painful conditions.

Because of adverse eye findings in animal studies with drugs of this class, it is recommended that ophthalmic studies be carried out if any change or disturbance in vision occurs.

Information for Patients:

Naproxen, like other drugs of its class, is not free of side effects. The side effects of these drugs can cause discomfort and, rarely, there are more serious side effects, such as gastrointestinal bleeding, which may result in hospitalization and even fatal outcomes.

NSAIDs (Nonsteroidal Anti-Inflammatory Drugs) are often essential agents in the management of arthritis and have a major role in the treatment of pain, but they also may be commonly employed for conditions which are less serious.

Physicians may wish to discuss with their patients the potential risks (see Warnings, Precautions, and Adverse Reactions sections) and likely benefits of NSAID treatment, particularly when the drugs are used for less serious conditions where treatment without NSAIDs may represent an acceptable alternative to both the patient and physician.

Caution should be exercised by patients whose activities require alertness if they experience drowsiness, dizziness, vertigo or depression during therapy with the drug.

Laboratory Tests:

Because serious GI tract ulceration and bleeding can occur without warning symptoms, physicians should follow chronically treated patients for the signs and symptoms of ulceration and bleeding and should inform them of the importance of this follow-up (see Risk of GI Ulceration, Bleeding and Perforation with NSAID Therapy).

Drug Interactions:

In vitro studies have shown that naproxen anion, because of its affinity for protein, may displace from their binding sites other drugs which are also albumin-bound. Theoretically, the naproxen anion itself could likewise be displaced. Short-term controlled studies failed to show that taking the drug significantly affects prothrombin times when administered to individuals on coumarin-type anticoagulants. Caution is advised nonetheless, since interactions have been seen with other nonsteroidal agents of this class. Similarly, patients receiving the drug and a hydantoin, sulfonamide or sulfonylurea should be observed for signs of toxicity to these drugs.

The natriuretic effect of furosemide has been reported to be inhibited by some drugs of this class. Inhibition of renal lithium clearance leading to increases in plasma lithium concentrations has also been reported

This and other nonsteroidal anti-inflammatory drugs can reduce the antihypertensive effect of propranolol and other beta-blockers.

Probenecid given concurrently increases naproxen anion plasma levels and extends its plasma half-life significantly.

Caution should be used if this drug is administered concomitantly with methotrexate. Naproxen and other nonsteroidal anti-inflammatory drugs have been reported to reduce the tubular secretion of methotrexate in an animal model, possibly enhancing the toxicity of that drug.

Drug/Laboratory Test Interactions:

The drug may decrease platelet aggregation and prolong bleeding time. This effect should be kept in mind when bleeding times are determined.

The administration of the drug may result in increased urinary values for 17-ketogenic steroids because of an interaction between the drug and/or its metabolites with m-dinitrobenzene used in this assay. Although 17-hydroxy-corticosteroid measurements (Porter-Silber test) do not appear to be artifactually altered, it is suggested that therapy with the drug be temporarily discontinued 72 hours before adrenal function tests are performed.

The drug may interfere with some urinary assays of 5-hydroxy indoleacetic acid (5HIAA).

Carcinogenesis:

A two-year study was performed in rats to evaluate the carcinogenic potential of the drug. No evidence of carcinogenicity was found.

Pregnancy:

Teratogenic Effects: Pregnancy Category B. Reproduction studies have been performed in rats, rabbits and mice at doses up to 6 times the human dose and have revealed no evidence of impaired fertility or harm to the fetus due to the drug. There are, however, no adequate and well-controlled studies in pregnant women. Because animal reproduction studies are not always predictive of human response, the drug should not be used during pregnancy unless clearly needed. Because of the known effect of drugs of this class on the human fetal cardiovascular system (closure of ductus arteriosus), use during late pregnancy should be avoided.

Non-teratogenic Effects: As with other drugs known to inhibit prostaglandin synthesis, an increased incidence of dystocia and delayed parturition occurred in rats.

Nursing Mothers:

The naproxen anion has been found in the milk of lactating women at a concentration of approximately 1% of that found in the plasma. Because of the possible adverse effects of prostaglandin-inhibiting drugs on neonates, use in nursing mothers should be avoided.

Pediatric Use:

Safety and effectiveness in children below the age of 2 years have not been established. Pediatric dosing recommendations for juvenile arthritis are based on well-controlled studies (see Dosage and Administration). There are no adequate effectiveness or dose-response data for other pediatric conditions, but the experience in juvenile arthritis and other use experience have established that single doses of 2.5-5 mg/kg, with total daily dose not exceeding 15 mg/kg/day, are safe in children over 2 years of age.

ADVERSE REACTIONS

The following adverse reactions are divided into 3 parts based on frequency and likelihood of causal relationship to naproxen.

Incidence greater than 1%

Probable Causal Relationship:

Adverse reactions reported in controlled clinical trials in 960 patients treated for rheu-

Central Nervous System: Depression, dream abnormalities, inability to concentrate, insomnia, malaise, myalgia and muscle weakness.

Dermatologic: Alopecia, photosensitive dermatitis, skin rashes.

Special Senses: Hearing impairment.

Cardiovascular: Congestive heart failure.

Respiratory: Eosinophilic pneumonitis.

General: Anaphylactoid reactions, menstrual disorders, pyrexia (chills and fever).

Causal Relationship Unknown:

Other reactions have been reported in circumstances in which a causal relationship could not be established. However, in these rarely reported events, the possibility cannot be excluded. Therefore, these observations are being listed to serve as alerting information to the physicians:

Hematologic: Aplastic anemia, hemolytic anemia.

Central Nervous System: Aseptic meningitis, cognitive dysfunction.

Dermatologic: Epidermal necrolysis, erythema multiforme, photosensitivity reactions resembling porphyria cutanea tarda and epidermolysis bullosa, Stevens-Johnson syndrome, urticaria.

Gastrointestinal: Non-peptic gastrointestinal ulceration, ulcerative stomatitis.

Cardiovascular: Vasculitis.

General: Angioneurotic edema, hyperglycemia, hypoglycemia.

OVERDOSAGE

Significant overdosage may be characterized by drowsiness, heartburn, indigestion, nausea or vomiting. A few patients have experienced seizures, but it is not clear whether or not these were drug related. It is not known what dose of the drug would be life threatening. The oral LD_{50} of the drug is 543 mg/kg in rats, 1,234 mg/kg in mice, 4,110 mg/kg in hamsters and greater than 1,000 mg/kg in dogs.

Should a patient ingest a large number of tablets or a large volume of suspension, accidentally or purposefully, the stomach may be emptied and usual supportive measures employed. In animals 0.5 g/kg of activated charcoal was effective in reducing plasma levels of naproxen. Hemodialysis does not decrease the plasma concentration of naproxen because of the high degree of its protein binding.

DOSAGE AND ADMINISTRATION

A measuring cup marked in 1/2 teaspoon and 2.5 milliliter increments is provided with the suspension. This cup or a teaspoon may be used to measure the appropriate dose.

For Rheumatoid Arthritis, Osteoarthritis, and Ankylosing Spondylitis:

The recommended dose of NAPROSYN® (naproxen) in adults is 250 mg (10 mL or 2 tsp of suspension), 375 mg (15 mL or 3 tsp), or 500 mg (20 mL or 4 tsp) twice daily (morning and evening). During long-term administration, the dose may be adjusted up or down depending on the clinical response of the patient. A lower daily dose may suffice for long-term administration. The morning and evening doses do not have to be equal in size and the administration of the drug more frequently than twice daily is not necessary. In patients who tolerate lower doses well, the dose may be increased to 1,500 mg per day for limited periods when a higher level of anti-inflammatory/analgesic activity is required. When treating such patients with the 1,500 mg/day dose, the physician should observe sufficient increased clinical benefits to offset the potential increased risk (see Clinical Pharmacology).

Symptomatic improvement in arthritis usually begins within 2 weeks. However, if improvement is not seen within this period, a trial for an additional 2 weeks should be considered.

For Juvenile Arthritis:

The recommended total daily dose of NAPROSYN is approximately 10 mg/kg given in 2 divided doses. One-half of the 250 mg tablet may be used to approximate this dose. The following table may be used as a guide for the suspension:

Child's Weight	Dose
13 kg (29 lb)	2.5 mL (1/2 tsp) b.i.d.
25 kg (55 lb)	5 mL (1 tsp) b.i.d.
38 kg (84 lb)	7.5 mL (1-1/2 tsp) b.i.d.

matoid arthritis or osteoarthritis are listed below. In general, these reactions were reported 2 to 10 times more frequently than they were in studies in the 962 patients treated for mild to moderate pain or for dysmenorrhea.

A clinical study found gastrointestinal reactions to be more frequent and more severe in rheumatoid arthritis patients taking 1,500 mg naproxen daily compared to those taking 750 mg daily (see Clinical Pharmacology).

In controlled clinical trials with about 80 children and in well-monitored open studies with about 400 children with juvenile arthritis, the incidences of rash and prolonged bleeding times were increased, the incidences of gastrointestinal and central nervous system reactions were about the same, and the incidences of other reactions were lower in children than in adults.

Gastrointestinal: The most frequent complaints reported related to the gastrointestinal tract. They were: constipation*, heartburn*, abdominal pain*, nausea*, dyspepsia, diarrhea, stomatitis.

Central Nervous System: Headache*, dizziness*, drowsiness*, lightheadedness, vertigo.

Dermatologic: Itching (pruritus)*, skin eruptions*, ecchymoses*, sweating, purpura.

Special Senses: Tinnitus*, hearing disturbances, visual disturbances.

Cardiovascular: Edema*, dyspnea*, palpitations.

General: Thirst.

*Incidence of reported reaction between 3% and 9%. Those reactions occurring in less than 3% of the patients are unmarked.

Incidence less than 1%

Probable Causal Relationship:
The following adverse reactions were reported less frequently than 1% during controlled clinical trials and through voluntary reports since marketing. The probability of a causal relationship exists between the drug and these adverse reactions:

Gastrointestinal: Abnormal liver function tests, colitis, gastrointestinal bleeding and/or perforation, hematemesis, jaundice, melena, peptic ulceration with bleeding and/or perforation, vomiting.

Renal: Glomerular nephritis, hematuria, hyperkalemia, interstitial nephritis, nephrotic syndrome, renal disease, renal failure, renal papillary necrosis.

Hematologic: Agranulocytosis, eosinophilia, granulocytopenia, leukopenia, thrombocytopenia.

For Acute Gout:
The recommended starting dose of NAPROSYN is 750 mg (30 mL or 6 tsp), followed by 250 mg (10 mL or 2 tsp) every 8 hours until the attack has subsided.

For Mild to Moderate Pain, Primary Dysmenorrhea and Acute Tendinitis and Bursitis:
The recommended starting dose of NAPROSYN is 500 mg (20 mL or 4 tsp), followed by 250 mg (10 mL or 2 tsp) every 6 to 8 hours as required. The total daily dose should not exceed 1,250 mg (50 mL or 10 tsp).

HOW SUPPLIED

NAPROSYN® (naproxen) is available as yellow 250 mg tablets in light-resistant bottles of 100 tablets (NDC 18393-272-42) (NSN 6505-01-026-9730) and 500 tablets (NDC 18393-272-62) (NSN 6505-01-046-0126) or in cartons of 100 individually blister-packed tablets (NDC 18393-272-53) (NSN 6505-01-097-9611). Peach 375 mg tablets are available in light-resistant bottles of 100 tablets (NDC 18393-273-42) (NSN 6505-01-135-8462) and 500 tablets (NDC 18393-273-62) (NSN 6505-01-204-5297) or in cartons of 100 individually blister-packed tablets (NDC 18393-273-53) (NSN 6505-01-204-5298). Yellow 500 mg tablets are available in light-resistant bottles of 100 tablets (NDC 18393-277-42) (NSN 6505-01-200-2474) and 500 tablets (NDC 18393-277-62) (NSN 6505-01-186-8758) or in cartons of 100 individually blister-packed tablets (NDC 18393-277-53). Store at room temperature in well-closed containers; dispense in light-resistant containers.

NAPROSYN® suspension is available in 1 pint (474 mL) light-resistant bottles (NDC 18393-278-20). Measuring cups are provided so that one can be dispensed with each prescription. Store at room temperature; avoid excessive heat, above 40°C (104° F). Dispense in light-resistant container.

CAUTION: Federal law prohibits dispensing without prescription.

U.S. Patent Nos. 3,904,682; 3,998,966 and others.

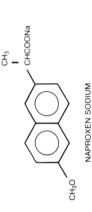

SYNTEX PUERTO RICO, INC.
HUMACAO, P.R. 00661

REVISED SEPTEMBER 1990
© 1990 SYNTEX PUERTO RICO, INC.
02-0273-53-02

ANAPROX®/ANAPROX® DS
(naproxen sodium)
Tablets

DESCRIPTION

ANAPROX® (naproxen sodium) filmcoated tablets for oral administration each contain 275 mg of naproxen sodium, which is equivalent to 250 mg naproxen with 25 mg (about 1 mEq) sodium. ANAPROX® DS (naproxen sodium) filmcoated tablets for oral administration each contain 550 mg of naproxen sodium, which is equivalent to 500 mg naproxen with 50 mg (about 2 mEq) sodium. Naproxen sodium is a member of the arylacetic acid group of nonsteroidal anti-inflammatory drugs.

The chemical name of naproxen sodium is 2-naphthaleneacetic acid, 6-methoxy-α-methyl-, sodium salt,(−)-. It has the following structure:

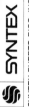

NAPROXEN SODIUM

Naproxen sodium is a white to creamy white, crystalline solid, freely soluble in water. Each ANAPROX 275 mg tablet contains naproxen sodium, the active ingredient; with lactose, magnesium stearate, and microcrystalline cellulose. The coating suspension may contain hydroxypropyl methylcellulose 2910, Opaspray K-1-4210A, polyethylene glycol 8000 or Opadry YS-1-4215. Each ANAPROX DS 550 mg tablet contains naproxen sodium, the active ingredient, with magnesium stearate, microcrystalline cellulose, povidone, and talc. The coating suspension may contain hydroxypropyl methylcellulose 2910, Opaspray K-1-4227, polyethylene glycol 8000 or Opadry YS-1-4216.

CLINICAL PHARMACOLOGY

The sodium salt of naproxen has been developed as an analgesic because it is more rapidly absorbed. Naproxen is a nonsteroidal anti-inflammatory drug with analgesic and antipyretic properties. Naproxen anion inhibits prostaglandin synthesis but beyond this its mode of action is unknown.

Naproxen sodium is rapidly and completely absorbed from the gastrointestinal tract. After administration of naproxen sodium, peak plasma levels of naproxen anion are attained at 1-2 hours with steady-state conditions normally achieved after 4-5 doses. The mean biological half-life of the anion in humans is approximately 13 hours, and at therapeutic levels it is greater than 99% albumin bound. Approximately 95% of the dose is excreted in the urine, primarily as naproxen, 6-0-desmethyl naproxen or their conjugates. The rate of excretion has been found to coincide closely with the rate of drug disappearance from the plasma. The drug does not induce metabolizing enzymes.

In children of 5 to 16 years of age with arthritis, plasma naproxen levels following a 5 mg/kg single dose of naproxen suspension (see Dosage and Administration) were found to be similar to those found in normal adults following a 500 mg dose. The terminal half-life appears to be similar in children and adults. Pharmacokinetic studies of naproxen were not performed in children of less than 5 years of age.

The drug was studied in patients with mild to moderate pain, and pain relief was obtained within 1 hour. It is not a narcotic and is not a CNS-acting drug. Controlled double-blind studies have demonstrated the analgesic properties of the drug in, for example, post-operative, post-partum, orthopedic and uterine contraction pain and dysmenorrhea. In dysmenorrheic patients, the drug reduces the level of prostaglandins in the uterus, which correlates with a reduction in the frequency and severity of uterine contractions. Analgesic action has been shown by such measures as reduction of pain intensity scores, increase in pain relief scores, decrease in numbers of patients requiring additional analgesic medication, and delay in time for required remedication. The analgesic effect has been found to last for up to 7 hours.

The drug was studied in patients with rheumatoid arthritis, osteoarthritis, juvenile arthritis, ankylosing spondylitis, tendinitis and bursitis, and acute gout. It is not a corticosteroid. Improvement in patients treated for rheumatoid arthritis has been demonstrated by a reduction in joint swelling, a reduction in pain, a reduction in duration of morning stiffness, a reduction in disease activity as assessed by both the investigator and patient, and by increased mobility as demonstrated by a reduction in walking time.

In patients with osteoarthritis, the therapeutic action of the drug has been shown by a reduction in joint pain or tenderness, an increase in range of motion in knee joints, increased mobility as demonstrated by a reduction in walking time, and improvement in capacity to perform activities of daily living impaired by the disease.

In clinical studies in patients with rheumatoid arthritis, osteoarthritis, and juvenile arthritis, the drug has been shown to be comparable to aspirin and indomethacin in controlling the aforementioned measures of disease activity, but the frequency and severity of the milder gastrointestinal adverse effects (nausea, dyspepsia, heartburn) and nervous system adverse effects (tinnitus, dizziness, lightheadedness) were less than in both the aspirin- and indomethacin-treated patients. It is not known whether the drug causes less peptic ulceration than aspirin.

In patients with ankylosing spondylitis, the drug has been shown to decrease night pain, morning stiffness and pain at rest. In double-blind studies the drug was shown to be as effective as aspirin, but with fewer side effects.

In patients with acute gout, a favorable response to the drug was shown by significant clearing of inflammatory changes (e.g., decrease in swelling, heat) within 24-48 hours, as well as by relief of pain and tenderness.

The drug may be used safely in combination with gold salts and/or corticosteroids; however, in controlled clinical trials, when added to the regimen of patients receiving corticosteroids it did not appear to cause greater improvement over that seen with corticosteroids alone. Whether the drug could be used in conjunction with partially effective doses of corticosteroid for a ''steroid-sparing'' effect has not been adequately studied. When added to the regimen of patients receiving gold salts, the drug did result in greater improvement. Its use in combination with salicylates is not recommended because data

Renal Effects: As with other nonsteroidal anti-inflammatory drugs, long-term administration of naproxen to animals has resulted in renal papillary necrosis and other abnormal renal pathology. In humans, there have been reports of acute interstitial nephritis with hematuria, proteinuria, and occasionally nephrotic syndrome.

A second form of renal toxicity has been seen in patients with prerenal conditions leading to a reduction in renal blood flow or blood volume, where the renal prostaglandins have a supportive role in the maintenance of renal perfusion. In these patients, administration of a nonsteroidal anti-inflammatory drug may cause a dose-dependent reduction in prostaglandin formation and may precipitate overt renal decompensation. Patients at greatest risk of this reaction are those with impaired renal function, heart failure, liver dysfunction, those taking diuretics, and the elderly. Discontinuation of nonsteroidal anti-inflammatory therapy is typically followed by recovery to the pretreatment state.

Naproxen sodium and its metabolites are eliminated primarily by the kidneys, therefore the drug should be used with great caution in patients with significantly impaired renal function and the monitoring of serum creatinine and/or creatinine clearance is advised in these patients. Caution should be used if the drug is given to patients with creatinine clearance of less than 20 mL/minute because accumulation of naproxen metabolites has been seen in such patients.

Chronic alcoholic liver disease and probably other forms of cirrhosis reduce the total plasma concentration of naproxen, but the plasma concentration of unbound naproxen is increased. Caution is advised when high doses are required and some adjustment of dosage may be required in these patients. It is prudent to use the lowest effective dose. Studies indicate that although total plasma concentration of naproxen is unchanged, the unbound plasma fraction of naproxen is increased in the elderly. Caution is advised when high doses are required and some adjustment of dosage may be required in elderly patients. As with other drugs used in the elderly, it is prudent to use the lowest effective dose.

As with other nonsteroidal anti-inflammatory drugs, borderline elevations of one or more liver tests may occur in up to 15% of patients. These abnormalities may progress, may remain essentially unchanged, or may be transient with continued therapy. The SGPT (ALT) test is probably the most sensitive indicator of liver dysfunction. Meaningful (3 times the upper limit of normal) elevations of SGPT or SGOT (AST) occurred in controlled clinical trials in less than 1% of patients. A patient with symptoms and/or signs suggesting liver dysfunction, or in whom an abnormal liver test has occurred, should be evaluated for evidence of the development of more severe hepatic reaction while on therapy with this drug. Severe hepatic reactions, including jaundice and cases of fatal hepatitis, have been reported with this drug as with other nonsteroidal anti-inflammatory drugs. Although such reactions are rare, if abnormal liver tests persist or worsen, if clinical signs and symptoms consistent with liver disease develop, or if systemic manifestations occur (e.g., eosinophilia, rash, etc.), this drug should be discontinued.

If steroid dosage is reduced or eliminated during therapy, the steroid dosage should be reduced slowly and the patients must be observed closely for any evidence of adverse effects, including adrenal insufficiency and exacerbation of symptoms of arthritis.

Patients with initial hemoglobin values of 10 grams or less who are to receive long-term therapy should have hemoglobin values determined periodically.

Peripheral edema has been observed in some patients. Since each naproxen sodium tablet contains approximately 25 mg or 50 mg (about 1 or 2 mEq) of sodium, this should be considered in patients whose overall intake of sodium must be markedly restricted. For these reasons, the drug should be used with caution in patients with fluid retention, hypertension or heart failure.

The antipyretic and anti-inflammatory activities of the drug may reduce fever and inflammation, thus diminishing their utility as diagnostic signs in detecting complications of presumed non-infectious, non-inflammatory painful conditions.

Because of adverse eye findings in animal studies with drugs of this class it is recommended that ophthalmic studies be carried out if any change or disturbance in vision occurs.

Information for Patients:

Naproxen sodium, like other drugs of its class, is not free of side effects. The side effects of these drugs can cause discomfort and, rarely, there are more serious side effects, such as gastrointestinal bleeding, which may result in hospitalization and even fatal outcomes.

are inadequate to demonstrate that the drug produces greater improvement over that achieved with aspirin alone. Further, there is some evidence that aspirin increases the rate of excretion of the drug.

Generally, improvement due to the drug has not been found to be dependent on age, sex, severity or duration of disease.

In clinical trials in patients with osteoarthritis and rheumatoid arthritis comparing treatments of 825 mg per day with 1,650 mg per day, there were trends toward increased efficacy with the higher dose and a more clearcut increase in adverse reactions, particularly gastrointestinal reactions severe enough to cause the patient to leave the trial, which approximately doubled.

In ^{51}Cr blood loss and gastroscopy studies with normal volunteers, daily administration of 1,100 mg of naproxen sodium has been demonstrated to cause statistically significantly less gastric bleeding and erosion than 3,250 mg of aspirin.

INDICATIONS AND USAGE

Naproxen sodium is indicated in the relief of mild to moderate pain and for the treatment of primary dysmenorrhea.

It is also indicated for the treatment of rheumatoid arthritis, osteoarthritis, juvenile arthritis, ankylosing spondylitis, tendinitis and bursitis, and acute gout.

CONTRAINDICATIONS

The drug is contraindicated in patients who have had allergic reactions to ANAPROX® (naproxen sodium), ANAPROX® DS or to NAPROSYN® (naproxen). It is also contraindicated in patients in whom aspirin or other nonsteroidal anti-inflammatory/analgesic drugs induce the syndrome of asthma, rhinitis, and nasal polyps. Both types of reactions have the potential of being fatal. Anaphylactoid reactions to ANAPROX, ANAPROX DS or NAPROSYN, whether of the true allergic type or the pharmacologic idiosyncratic (e.g., aspirin syndrome) type, usually but not always occur in patients with a known history of such reactions. Therefore, careful questioning of patients for such things as asthma, nasal polyps, urticaria, and hypotension associated with nonsteroidal anti-inflammatory drugs before starting therapy is important. In addition, if such symptoms occur during therapy, treatment should be discontinued.

WARNINGS

Risk of GI Ulceration, Bleeding and Perforation with NSAID Therapy:

Serious gastrointestinal toxicity such as bleeding, ulceration, and perforation, can occur at any time, with or without warning symptoms, in patients treated chronically with NSAID therapy. Although minor upper gastrointestinal problems, such as dyspepsia, are common, usually developing early in therapy, physicians should remain alert for ulceration and bleeding in patients treated chronically with NSAIDs even in the absence of previous GI tract symptoms. In patients observed in clinical trials of several months to two years' duration, symptomatic upper GI ulcers, gross bleeding or perforation appear to occur in approximately 1% of patients treated for 3-6 months, and in about 2-4% of patients treated for one year. Physicians should inform patients about the signs and/or symptoms of serious GI toxicity and what steps to take if they occur.

Studies to date have not identified any subset of patients not at risk of developing peptic ulceration and bleeding. Except for a prior history of serious GI events and other risk factors known to be associated with peptic ulcer disease, such as alcoholism, smoking, etc., no risk factors (e.g., age, sex) have been associated with increased risk. Elderly or debilitated patients seem to tolerate ulceration or bleeding less well than other individuals and most spontaneous reports of fatal GI events are in this population. Studies to date are inconclusive concerning the relative risk of various NSAIDs in causing such reactions. High doses of any NSAID probably carry a greater risk of these reactions, although controlled clinical trials showing this do not exist in most cases. In considering the use of relatively large doses (within the recommended dosage range), sufficient benefit should be anticipated to offset the potential increased risk of GI toxicity.

PRECAUTIONS

General:

ANAPROX (NAPROXEN SODIUM) OR ANAPROX DS (NAPROXEN SODIUM) SHOULD NOT BE USED CONCOMITANTLY WITH THE RELATED DRUG NAPROSYN (NAPROXEN) SINCE THEY BOTH CIRCULATE IN PLASMA AS THE NAPROXEN ANION.

NSAIDs (Nonsteroidal Anti-Inflammatory Drugs) are often essential agents in the management of arthritis and have a major role in the treatment of pain, but they also may be commonly employed for conditions which are less serious.

Physicians may wish to discuss with their patients the potential risks (see Warnings, Precautions, and Adverse Reactions sections) and likely benefits of NSAID treatment, particularly when the drugs are used for less serious conditions where treatment without NSAIDs may represent an acceptable alternative to both the patient and physician.

Caution should be exercised by patients whose activities require alertness if they experience drowsiness, dizziness, vertigo or depression during therapy with the drug.

Laboratory Tests:

Because serious GI tract ulceration and bleeding can occur without warning symptoms, physicians should follow chronically treated patients for the signs and symptoms of ulceration and bleeding and should inform them of the importance of this follow-up (see Risk of GI Ulcerations, Bleeding and Perforation with NSAID Therapy).

Drug Interactions:

In vitro studies have shown that naproxen anion, because of its affinity for protein, may displace from their binding sites other drugs which are also albumin-bound. Theoretically, the naproxen anion itself could likewise be displaced. Short-term controlled studies failed to show that taking the drug significantly affects prothrombin times when administered to individuals on coumarin-type anticoagulants. Caution is advised nonetheless, since interactions have been seen with other nonsteroidal agents of this class. Similarly, patients receiving the drug and a hydantoin, sulfonamide or sulfonylurea should be observed for signs of toxicity to these drugs.

The natriuretic effect of furosemide has been reported to be inhibited by some drugs of this class. Inhibition of renal lithium clearance leading to increases in plasma lithium concentrations has also been reported.

This and other nonsteroidal anti-inflammatory drugs can reduce the antihypertensive effect of propranolol and other beta-blockers.

Probenecid given concomitantly increases naproxen anion plasma levels and extends its plasma half-life significantly.

Caution should be used if this drug is administered concomitantly with methotrexate. Naproxen and other nonsteroidal anti-inflammatory drugs have been reported to reduce the tubular secretion of methotrexate in an animal model, possibly enhancing the toxicity of that drug.

Drug/Laboratory Test Interactions:

The drug may decrease platelet aggregation and prolong bleeding time. This effect should be kept in mind when bleeding times are determined.

The administration of the drug may result in increased urinary values for 17-ketogenic steroids because of an interaction between the drug and/or its metabolites with m-dinitrobenzene used in this assay. Although 17-hydroxy-corticosteroid measurements (Porter-Silber test) do not appear to be artifactually altered, it is suggested that therapy with the drug be temporarily discontinued 72 hours before adrenal function tests are performed.

The drug may interfere with some urinary assays of 5-hydroxy indoleacetic acid (5HIAA).

Carcinogenesis:

A two-year study was performed in rats to evaluate the carcinogenic potential of the drug. No evidence of carcinogenicity was found.

Pregnancy:

Teratogenic Effects: Pregnancy Category B. Reproduction studies have been performed in rats, rabbits and mice at doses up to six times the human dose and have revealed no evidence of impaired fertility or harm to the fetus due to the drug. There are, however, no adequate and well-controlled studies in pregnant women. Because animal reproduction studies are not always predictive of human response, the drug should not be used during pregnancy unless clearly needed. Because of the known effect of drugs of this class on the human fetal cardiovascular system (closure of ductus arteriosus), use during late pregnancy should be avoided.

Non-teratogenic Effects: As with other drugs known to inhibit prostaglandin synthesis, an increased incidence of dystocia and delayed parturition occurred in rats

Nursing Mothers:

The naproxen anion has been found in the milk of lactating women at a concentration of approximately 1% of that found in the plasma. Because of the possible adverse effects of prostaglandin-inhibiting drugs on neonates, use in nursing mothers should be avoided.

Pediatric Use:

Safety and effectiveness in children below the age of 2 years have not been established. Pediatric dosing recommendations for juvenile arthritis are based on well-controlled studies. There are no adequate effectiveness or dose-response data for other pediatric conditions, but the experience in juvenile arthritis and other use experience have established that single doses of 2.5-5 mg/kg (as naproxen suspension, see Dosage and Administration), with total daily dose not exceeding 15 mg/kg/day, are safe in children over 2 years of age.

ADVERSE REACTIONS

The following adverse reactions are divided into three parts based on frequency and likelihood of causal relationship to naproxen sodium.

Incidence greater than 1%

Probable Causal Relationship:

Adverse reactions reported in controlled clinical trials in 960 patients treated for rheumatoid arthritis or osteoarthritis are listed below. In general, these reactions were reported 2 to 10 times more frequently than they were in studies in the 962 patients treated for mild to moderate pain or for dysmenorrhea.

A clinical study found gastrointestinal reactions to be more frequent and more severe in rheumatoid arthritis patients taking 1,650 mg naproxen sodium daily compared to those taking 825 mg daily (see Clinical Pharmacology).

In controlled clinical trials with about 80 children and in well monitored open studies with about 400 children with juvenile arthritis, the incidences of rash and prolonged bleeding times were increased, the incidences of gastrointestinal and central nervous system reactions were about the same, and the incidences of other reactions were lower in children than in adults.

Gastrointestinal: The most frequent complaints reported related to the gastrointestinal tract. They were: constipation*, heartburn*, abdominal pain*, nausea*, dyspepsia, diarrhea, stomatitis.

Central Nervous System: Headache*, dizziness*, drowsiness*, lightheadedness, vertigo.

Dermatologic: Itching (pruritus)*, skin eruptions*, ecchymoses*, sweating, purpura.

Special Senses: Tinnitus*, hearing disturbances, visual disturbances.

Cardiovascular: Edema*, dyspnea*, palpitations.

General: Thirst.

*Incidence of reported reaction between 3% and 9%. Those reactions occurring in less than 3% of the patients are unmarked.

Incidence less than 1%

Probable Causal Relationship:

The following adverse reactions were reported less frequently than 1% during controlled clinical trials and through voluntary reports since marketing. The probability of a causal relationship exists between the drug and these adverse reactions.

Gastrointestinal: Abnormal liver function tests, colitis, gastrointestinal bleeding and/or perforation, hematemesis, jaundice, melena, peptic ulceration with bleeding and/or perforation, vomiting.

Renal: Glomerular nephritis, hematuria, hyperkalemia, interstitial nephritis, nephrotic syndrome, renal disease, renal failure, renal papillary necrosis.

Hematologic: Agranulocytosis, eosinophilia, granulocytopenia, leukopenia, thrombocytopenia.

Central Nervous System: Depression, dream abnormalities, inability to concentrate, insomnia, malaise, myalgia and muscle weakness.

Dermatologic: Alopecia, photosensitive dermatitis, skin rashes.

Special Senses: Hearing impairment.

resembling porphyria cutanea tarda and epidermolysis bullosa, Stevens-Johnson syndrome, urticaria.

Gastrointestinal: Non-peptic gastrointestinal ulceration, ulcerative stomatitis.

Cardiovascular: Vasculitis.

General: Angioneurotic edema, hyperglycemia, hypoglycemia.

OVERDOSAGE

Significant overdosage may be characterized by drowsiness, heartburn, indigestion, nausea or vomiting. Because naproxen sodium may be rapidly absorbed, high and early blood levels should be anticipated. A few patients have experienced seizures, but it is not clear whether or not these were drug related. It is not known what dose of the drug would be life threatening. The oral LD_{50} of the drug is 543 mg/kg in rats, 1,234 mg/kg in mice, 4,110 mg/kg in hamsters and greater than 1,000 mg/kg in dogs.

Should a patient ingest a large number of tablets, accidentally or purposefully, the stomach may be emptied and usual supportive measures employed. In animals 0.5 g/kg of activated charcoal was effective in reducing plasma levels of naproxen. Hemodialysis does not decrease the plasma concentration of naproxen because of the high degree of its protein binding.

DOSAGE AND ADMINISTRATION

For Mild to Moderate Pain, Primary Dysmenorrhea and Acute Tendinitis and Bursitis:

The recommended starting dose is 550 mg, followed by 275 mg every 6 to 8 hours, as required. The total daily dose should not exceed 1,375 mg.

For Rheumatoid Arthritis, Osteoarthritis, and Ankylosing Spondylitis:

The recommended dose in adults is 275 mg or 550 mg twice daily (morning and evening). During long-term administration, the dose may be adjusted up or down depending on the clinical response of the patient. A lower daily dose may suffice for long-term administration. The morning and evening doses do not have to be equal in size and the administration of the drug more frequently than twice daily is not necessary.

In patients who tolerate lower doses well, the dose may be increased to 1,650 mg per day for limited periods when a higher level of anti-inflammatory/analgesic activity is required. When treating such patients with the 1,650 mg/day dose, the physician should observe sufficient increased clinical benefits to offset the potential increased risk (see Clinical Pharmacology).

Symptomatic improvement in arthritis usually begins within two weeks. However, if improvement is not seen within this period, a trial for an additional two weeks should be considered.

For Acute Gout:

The recommended starting dose is 825 mg, followed by 275 mg every eight hours until the attack has subsided.

For Juvenile Arthritis:

The recommended total daily dose is approximately 10 mg/kg given in two divided doses. The 275 mg ANAPROX tablet is not well suited to this dosage so use of the related drug NAPROSYN® (naproxen) as the 250 mg scored tablet or the 125 mg/5 mL suspension is recommended for this indication.

HOW SUPPLIED

ANAPROX® (naproxen sodium) is available in filmcoated tablets of 275 mg (light blue), in bottles of 100 tablets (NDC 18393-274-42) (NSN 6505-01-155-5157) and 500 tablets (NDC 18393-274-62) (NSN 6505-01-130-6832) or in cartons of 100 individually blister packed tablets (NDC 18393-274-53). ANAPROX® DS (naproxen sodium) is available in filmcoated tablets of 550 mg (dark blue), in bottles of 100 tablets (NDC 18393-276-42) (NSN 6505-01-305-8174) and 500 tablets (NDC 18393-276-62) or in cartons of 100 individually blister packed tablets (NDC 18393-276-53). Store at room temperature in well-closed containers.

CAUTION: Federal law prohibits dispensing without prescription.

U.S. Patent Nos. 4,009,197; 3,998,966 and others.

Cardiovascular: Congestive heart failure.

Respiratory: Eosinophilic pneumonitis.

General: Anaphylactoid reactions, menstrual disorders, pyrexia (chills and fever).

Causal Relationship Unknown:

Other reactions have been reported in circumstances in which a causal relationship could not be established. However, in these rarely reported events, the possibility cannot be excluded. Therefore these observations are being listed to serve as alerting information to the physicians.

Hematologic: Aplastic anemia, hemolytic anemia.

Central Nervous System: Aseptic meningitis, cognitive dysfunction.

Dermatologic: Epidermal necrolysis, erythema multiforme, photosensitivity reactions

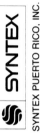

SYNTEX

SYNTEX PUERTO RICO, INC.
HUMACAO, P.R. 00661

REVISED SEPTEMBER 1990
© 1990 SYNTEX PUERTO RICO, INC.
D2-0276-42-04

SYNAREL® (nafarelin acetate)

Nasal Solution 2 mg/mL

(as nafarelin base)

DESCRIPTION

SYNAREL (nafarelin acetate) Nasal Solution is intended for administration as a spray to the nasal mucosa. Nafarelin acetate, the active component of SYNAREL Nasal Solution, is a decapeptide with the chemical name: 5-oxo-L-prolyl-L-histidyl-L-tryptophyl-L-seryl-L-tyrosyl-3-(2-naphthyl)-D-alanyl-L-leucyl-L-arginyl-L-prolyl-glycinamide acetate. Nafarelin acetate is a synthetic analog of the naturally occurring gonadotropin-releasing hormone (GnRH).

Nafarelin acetate has the following chemical structure:

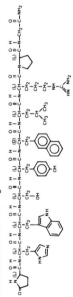

SYNAREL Nasal Solution contains nafarelin acetate (2 mg/mL, content expressed as nafarelin base) in a solution of benzalkonium chloride, glacial acetic acid, sodium hydroxide or hydrochloric acid (to adjust pH), sorbitol, and purified water.

After priming the pump unit for SYNAREL, each actuation of the unit delivers approximately 100 μL of the spray containing approximately 200 μg nafarelin base. The contents of one spray bottle are intended to deliver at least 60 sprays.

CLINICAL PHARMACOLOGY

Nafarelin acetate is a potent agonistic analog of gonadotropin-releasing hormone (GnRH). At the onset of administration, nafarelin stimulates the release of the pituitary gonadotropins, LH and FSH, resulting in a temporary increase of ovarian steroidogenesis. Repeated dosing abolishes the stimulatory effect on the pituitary gland. Twice daily administration leads to decreased secretion of gonadal steroids by about 4 weeks; consequently, tissues and functions that depend on gonadal steroids for their maintenance become quiescent.

Nafarelin acetate is rapidly absorbed into the systemic circulation after intranasal administration. Maximum serum concentrations (measured by RIA) are achieved between 10 and 40 minutes. Following a single dose of 200 μg base, the observed average peak concentration is 0.6 ng/mL, whereas following a single dose of 400 μg base, the observed average peak concentration is 1.8 ng/mL. Bioavailability from a 400 μg dose averaged 2.8%. The average serum half-life of nafarelin following intranasal administration is approximately 3 hours. About 80% of nafarelin acetate is bound to plasma proteins at 4°C.

After subcutaneous administration of ^{14}C-nafarelin acetate, 44-55% of the dose was recovered in urine and 18.5-44.2% was recovered in feces. Approximately 3% of the administered dose appears as unchanged nafarelin in urine. The ^{14}C serum half-life of the metabolites is about 85.5 hours. Six metabolites of nafarelin have been identified of which the major metabolite is Tyr-D(2)-Nal-Leu-Arg-Pro-Gly-NH$_2$(5-10). The activity of the metabolites, the metabolism of nafarelin by nasal mucosa, and the pharmacokinetics of the drug in hepatic- and renal-impaired patients have not been determined.

The effect of rhinitis or a topical decongestant on SYNAREL has not been determined.

In controlled clinical studies, SYNAREL at doses of 400 and 800 μg/day for 6 months was shown to be comparable to danazol, 800 mg/day, in relieving the clinical symptoms of endometriosis (pelvic pain, dysmenorrhea, and dyspareunia) and in reducing the size of endometrial implants as determined by laparoscopy. The clinical significance of a decrease in endometriotic lesions is not known at this time and in addition, laparoscopic staging of endometriosis does not necessarily correlate with severity of symptoms.

SYNAREL 400 μg daily induced amenorrhea in approximately 65%, 80%, and 90% of the patients after 60, 90, and 120 days, respectively. In the first, second, and third post-treatment months, normal menstrual cycles resumed in 4%, 82%, and 100%, respectively, of those patients who did not become pregnant.

At the end of treatment, 60% of patients who received SYNAREL, 400 μg/day, were symptom free, 32% had mild symptoms, 7% had moderate symptoms and 1% had severe symptoms. Of the 60% of patients who had complete relief of symptoms at the end of treatment, 17% had moderate symptoms 6 months after treatment was discontinued, 33% had mild symptoms, 50% remained symptom free, and no patient had severe symptoms.

During the first two months use of SYNAREL, some women experience vaginal bleeding of variable duration and intensity. In all likelihood, this bleeding represents estrogen withdrawal bleeding, and is expected to stop spontaneously. If vaginal bleeding continues, the possibility of lack of compliance with the dosing regimen should be considered. If the patient is complying carefully with the regimen, an increase in dose to 400 μg twice a day should be considered.

There is no evidence that pregnancy rates are enhanced or adversely affected by the use of SYNAREL.

INDICATIONS AND USAGE

SYNAREL is indicated for management of endometriosis, including pain relief and reduction of endometriotic lesions. Experience with SYNAREL for the management of endometriosis has been limited to women 18 years of age and older treated for 6 months.

CONTRAINDICATIONS

1. Hypersensitivity to GnRH, GnRH agonist analogs or any of the excipients in SYNAREL;
2. Undiagnosed abnormal vaginal bleeding;
3. Use in pregnancy or in women who may become pregnant while receiving the drug. SYNAREL may cause fetal harm when administered to a pregnant woman. Major fetal abnormalities were observed in rats, but not in mice or rabbits after administration of SYNAREL throughout gestation. There was a dose-related increase in fetal mortality and a decrease in fetal weight in rats (see Pregnancy Section). The effects on rat fetal mortality are expected consequences of the alterations in hormonal levels brought about by the drug. If this drug is used during pregnancy or if the patient becomes pregnant while taking this drug, she should be apprised of the potential hazard to the fetus;
4. Use in women who are breast feeding (see Nursing Mothers Section).

WARNINGS

Safe use of nafarelin acetate in pregnancy has not been established clinically. Before starting treatment with SYNAREL, pregnancy must be excluded.

When used regularly at the recommended dose, SYNAREL usually inhibits ovulation and stops menstruation. Contraception is not insured, however, by taking SYNAREL, particularly if patients miss successive doses. Therefore, patients should use nonhormonal methods of contraception. Patients should be advised to see their physician if they believe they may be pregnant. If a patient becomes pregnant during treatment, the drug must be discontinued and the patient must be apprised of the potential risk to the fetus.

PRECAUTIONS

General

As with other drugs in this class, ovarian cysts have been reported to occur in the first two months of therapy with SYNAREL. Many, but not all, of these events occurred in patients with polycystic ovarian disease. These cystic enlargements may resolve spontaneously, generally by about four to six weeks of therapy, but in some cases may require discontinuation of drug and/or surgical intervention.

Information for Patients

An information pamphlet for patients is included with the product. Patients should be aware of the following information:

1. Since menstruation should stop with effective doses of SYNAREL, the patient should notify her physician if regular menstruation persists. The cause of vaginal spotting, bleeding or menstruation could be non-compliance with the treatment regimen, or it could be that a higher dose of the drug is required to achieve amenorrhea. The patient should be questioned regarding her compliance. If she is careful and compliant, and menstruation persists to the second month, consideration should be given to doubling the dose of SYNAREL. If the patient has missed several doses, she should be counseled on the importance of taking SYNAREL regularly as prescribed.

2. Patients should not use SYNAREL if they are pregnant, breast feeding, have undiagnosed abnormal vaginal bleeding, or are allergic to any of the ingredients in SYNAREL.

3. Safe use of the drug in pregnancy has not been established clinically. Therefore, a nonhormonal method of contraception should be used during treatment. Patients should be advised that if they miss successive doses of SYNAREL, breakthrough bleeding or ovulation may occur with the potential for conception. If a patient becomes pregnant during treatment, she should discontinue treatment and consult her physician.

4. Those adverse events occurring most frequently in clinical studies with SYNAREL are associated with hypoestrogenism; the most frequently reported are hot flashes, headaches, emotional lability, decreased libido, vaginal dryness, acne, myalgia, and reduction in breast size.

Nursing Mothers

It is not known whether SYNAREL is excreted in human milk. Because many drugs are excreted in human milk, and because the effects of SYNAREL on lactation and/or the breastfed child have not been determined, SYNAREL should not be used by nursing mothers.

Pediatric Use

Safety and effectiveness in children have not been established.

ADVERSE REACTIONS

As would be expected with a drug which lowers serum estradiol levels, the most frequently reported adverse reactions were those related to hypoestrogenism.

In controlled studies comparing SYNAREL (400 μg/day) and danazol (600 or 800 mg/day), adverse reactions most frequently reported and thought to be drug-related are shown in the figure below.

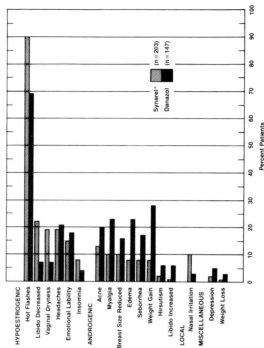

ADVERSE EVENTS DURING 6 MONTH TREATMENT WITH SYNAREL® 400 μg/day vs DANAZOL 600 OR 800 mg/day

In addition, less than 1% of patients experienced paresthesia, palpitations, chloasma, maculopapular rash, eye pain, urticaria, asthenia, lactation, breast engorgement, and arthralgia. In formal clinical trials, immediate hypersensitivity thought to be possibly or probably related to nafarelin occurred in 3 (0.2%) of 1509 healthy subjects or patients.

Changes in Bone Density

After six months of treatment with SYNAREL, vertebral trabecular bone density and total vertebral bone mass, measured by quantitative computed tomography (QCT), decreased by an average of 8.7% and 4.3%, respectively, compared to pretreatment levels. There was partial recovery of bone density in the post-treatment period; the average trabecular bone density and total bone mass were 4.9% and 3.3% less than the pretreatment levels, respectively. Total vertebral bone

Estrogen levels returned to normal after treatment was discontinued. Nasal irritation occurred in about 10% of all patients who used intranasal nafarelin.

5. The induced hypoestrogenic state results in a small loss in bone density over the course of treatment, some of which may not be reversible. During one six-month treatment period, this bone loss should not be important. In patients with major risk factors for decreased bone mineral content such as chronic alcohol and/or tobacco use, strong family history of osteoporosis, or chronic use of drugs that can reduce bone mass such as anticonvulsants or corticosteroids, SYNAREL therapy may pose an additional risk. In these patients the risks and benefits must be weighed carefully before therapy with SYNAREL is instituted. Repeated courses of treatment with gonadotropin-releasing hormone analogs are not advisable in patients with major risk factors for loss of bone mineral content.

6. Patients with intercurrent rhinitis should consult their physician for the use of a topical nasal decongestant. If the use of a topical nasal decongestant is required during treatment with SYNAREL, the decongestant must be used at least 30 minutes after SYNAREL dosing to decrease the possibility of reducing drug absorption.

7. Retreatment cannot be recommended since safety data beyond 6 months are not available.

Drug Interactions

No pharmacokinetic-based drug-drug interaction studies have been conducted with SYNAREL. However, because nafarelin acetate is a peptide that is primarily degraded by peptidase and not by cytochrome P-450 enzymes, and the drug is only about 80% bound to plasma proteins at 4°C, drug interactions would not be expected to occur.

Drug/Laboratory Test Interactions

Administration of SYNAREL in therapeutic doses results in suppression of the pituitary-gonadal system. Normal function is usually restored within 4 to 8 weeks after treatment is discontinued. Therefore, diagnostic tests of pituitary gonadotropic and gonadal functions conducted during treatment and up to 4 to 8 weeks after discontinuation of SYNAREL therapy may be misleading.

Carcinogenesis, Mutagenesis, Impairment of Fertility

Carcinogenicity studies of nafarelin were conducted in rats (24 months) at doses up to 100 µg/kg/day and mice (18 months) at doses up to 500 µg/kg/day using intramuscular doses (up to 110 times and 560 times the maximum recommended human intranasal dose, respectively). These multiples of the human dose are based on the relative bioavailability of the drug by the two routes of administration. As seen with other GnRH agonists, nafarelin acetate given to laboratory rodents at high doses for prolonged periods induced proliferative responses (hyperplasia and/or neoplasia) of endocrine organs. At 24 months, there was an increase in the incidence of pituitary tumors (adenoma/carcinoma) in high-dose female rats and a dose-related increase in male rats. There was an increase in pancreatic islet cell adenomas in both sexes, and in benign testicular and ovarian tumors in the treated groups. There was a dose-related increase in benign adrenal medullary tumors in treated female rats. In mice, there was a dose-related increase in Harderian gland tumors in males and an increase in pituitary adenomas in high-dose females. No metastases of these tumors were observed. It is known that tumorigenicity in rodents is particularly sensitive to hormonal stimulation.

Mutagenicity studies have been performed with nafarelin acetate using bacterial, yeast, and mammalian systems. These studies provided no evidence of mutagenic potential.

Reproduction studies in male and female rats have shown full reversibility of fertility suppression when drug treatment was discontinued after continuous administration for up to 6 months.

Pregnancy, Teratogenic Effects

Pregnancy Category X. See 'Contraindications.' Intramuscular SYNAREL® was administered to rats throughout gestation at 0.4, 1.6, and 6.4 µg/kg/day (about 0.5, 2, and 7 times the maximum recommended human intranasal dose based on the relative bioavailability by the two routes of administration). An increase in major fetal abnormalities was observed in 4/80 fetuses at the highest dose. A similar, repeat study at the same doses in rats and studies in mice and rabbits at doses up to 600 µg/kg/day and 0.18 µg/kg/day, respectively, failed to demonstrate an increase in fetal abnormalities after administration throughout gestation. In rats and rabbits, there was a dose-related increase in fetal mortality and a decrease in fetal weight with the highest dose.

mass, measured by dual photon absorptiometry (DPA), decreased by a mean of 5.9% at the end of treatment. Mean total vertebral mass, re-examined by DPA six months after completion of treatment, was 1.4% below pretreatment levels. There was little, if any, decrease in the mineral content in compact bone of the distal radius and second metacarpal. Use of SYNAREL for longer than the recommended six months or in the presence of other known risk factors for decreased bone mineral content may cause additional bone loss.

Changes in Laboratory Values During Treatment

Plasma enzymes. During clinical trials with SYNAREL, regular laboratory monitoring revealed that SGOT and SGPT levels were more than twice the upper limit of normal in only one patient each. There was no other clinical or laboratory evidence of abnormal liver function and levels returned to normal in both patients after treatment was stopped.

Lipids. At enrollment, 9% of the patients in the SYNAREL 400 µg/day group and 2% of the patients in the danazol group had total cholesterol values above 250 mg/dL. These patients also had cholesterol values above 250 mg/dL at the end of treatment.

Of those patients whose pretreatment cholesterol values were below 250 mg/dL, 6% in the SYNAREL group and 18% in the danazol group, had post-treatment values above 250 mg/dL.

The mean ($\pm$ SEM) pretreatment values for total cholesterol from all patients were 191.8 (4.3) mg/dL in the SYNAREL group and 193.1 (4.6) mg/dL in the danazol group. At the end of treatment, the mean values for total cholesterol from all patients were 204.5 (4.8) mg/dL in the SYNAREL group and 207.7 (5.1) mg/dL in the danazol group. These increases from the pretreatment values were statistically significant ($p<0.05$) in both groups.

Triglycerides were increased above the upper limit of 150 mg/dL in 12% of the patients who received SYNAREL and in 7% of the patients who received danazol.

At the end of treatment, no patients receiving SYNAREL had abnormally low HDL cholesterol fractions (less than 30 mg/dL) compared with 43% of patients receiving danazol. None of the patients receiving SYNAREL had abnormally high LDL cholesterol fractions (greater than 190 mg/dL) compared with 15% of those receiving danazol. There was no increase in the LDL/HDL ratio in patients receiving SYNAREL, but there was approximately a 2-fold increase in the LDL/HDL ratio in patients receiving danazol.

Other changes. In comparative studies, the following changes were seen in approximately 10% to 15% of patients. Treatment with SYNAREL was associated with elevations of plasma phosphorous and eosinophil counts, and decreases in serum calcium and WBC counts Danazol therapy was associated with an increase of hematocrit and WBC.

OVERDOSAGE

In experimental animals, a single subcutaneous administration of up to 60 times the recommended human dose (on a µg/kg basis, not adjusted for bioavailability) had no adverse effects. At present, there is no clinical evidence of adverse effects following overdosage of GnRH analogs.

Based on studies in monkeys, SYNAREL is not absorbed after oral administration.

DOSAGE AND ADMINISTRATION

For the management of endometriosis, the recommended daily dose of SYNAREL is 400 µg. This is achieved by one spray (200 µg) into one nostril in the morning and one spray into the other nostril in the evening. Treatment should be started between days 2 and 4 of the menstrual cycle.

In an occasional patient, the 400 µg daily dose may not produce amenorrhea. For these patients with persistent regular menstruation after 2 months of treatment, the dose of SYNAREL may be increased to 800 µg daily. The 800 µg dose is administered as one spray into each nostril in the morning (a total of two sprays) and again in the evening.

The recommended duration of administration is six months. Retreatment cannot be recommended since safety data for retreatment are not available. If the symptoms of endometriosis recur after a course of therapy, and further treatment with SYNAREL is contemplated, it is recommended that bone density be assessed before retreatment begins to ensure that values are within normal limits.

If the use of a topical nasal decongestant is necessary during treatment with SYNAREL, the decongestant should not be used until at least 30 minutes after SYNAREL dosing.

At 400 µg/day, a bottle of SYNAREL provides a 30-day (about 60 sprays) supply. If the daily dose is increased, increase the supply to the patient to ensure uninterrupted treatment for the recommended duration of therapy.

HOW SUPPLIED

Each 0.5 ounce bottle (NDC 0033-2260-40) contains 10 mL SYNAREL (nafarelin acetate) Nasal Solution 2 mg/mL (as nafarelin base), and is supplied with a metered spray pump that delivers 200 µg of nafarelin per spray. A dust cover and a leaflet of patient instructions are also included.

Store upright at room temperature. Avoid heat above 30°C (86°F). Protect from light Protect from freezing.

CAUTION: Federal law prohibits dispensing without prescription.

U.S. Patent No. 4,234,571.

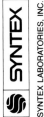 **SYNTEX**

SYNTEX LABORATORIES, INC.
PALO ALTO, CA 94304

REVISED APRIL 1991

© 1991 SYNTEX LABORATORIES, INC.
02-2260-40-03

SYNALAR®
(fluocinolone acetonide)
Cream 0.025%
for initiation of therapy in inflammatory dermatoses.
Cream 0.01%
for occlusive or maintenance therapy.

description

SYNALAR creams are intended for topical administration. The active component is the corticosteroid fluocinolone acetonide, which has the chemical name pregna-1,4-diene-3,20-dione,6,9-difluoro-11,21-dihydroxy-16,17-[(1-methylethylidene)bis (oxy)]-,(6α,11β,16α)-. It has the following chemical structure:

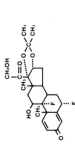

The creams contain fluocinolone acetonide 0.25 mg/g or 0.1 mg/g in a water-washable aqueous base of stearyl alcohol, propylene glycol, cetyl alcohol, polyoxyl 20 cetostearyl ether, mineral oil, white wax, simethicone, butylated hydroxytoluene, edetate disodium, citric acid, and purified water, with methylparaben and propylparaben as preservatives.

3. The treated skin area should not be bandaged or otherwise covered or wrapped as to be occlusive unless directed by the physician.
4. Patients should report any signs of local adverse reactions especially under occlusive dressing.
5. Parents of pediatric patients should be advised not to use tight-fitting diapers or plastic pants on a child being treated in the diaper area, as these garments may constitute occlusive dressings.

Laboratory Tests
The following tests may be helpful in evaluating the HPA axis suppression:
Urinary free cortisol test
ACTH stimulation test

Carcinogenesis, Mutagenesis, and Impairment of Fertility
Long-term animal studies have not been performed to evaluate the carcinogenic potential or the effect on fertility of topical corticosteroids.
Studies to determine mutagenicity with prednisolone and hydrocortisone have revealed negative results.

Pregnancy Category C
Corticosteroids are generally teratogenic in laboratory animals when administered systemically at relatively low dosage levels. The more potent corticosteroids have been shown to be teratogenic after dermal application in laboratory animals. There are no adequate and well-controlled studies in pregnant women on teratogenic effects from topically applied corticosteroids. Therefore, topical corticosteroids should be used during pregnancy only if the potential benefit justifies the potential risk to the fetus. Drugs of this class should not be used extensively on pregnant patients, in large amounts, or for prolonged periods of time.

Nursing Mothers
It is not known whether topical administration of corticosteroids could result in sufficient systemic absorption to produce detectable quantities in breast milk. Systemically administered corticosteroids are secreted into breast milk in quantities not likely to have a deleterious effect on the infant. Nevertheless, caution should be exercised when topical corticosteroids are administered to a nursing woman.

Pediatric Use
Pediatric patients may demonstrate greater susceptibility to topical corticosteroid-induced HPA axis suppression and Cushing's syndrome than mature patients because of a larger skin surface area to body weight ratio.
Hypothalamic-pituitary-adrenal (HPA) axis suppression, Cushing's syndrome, and intracranial hypertension have been reported in children receiving topical corticosteroids. Manifestations of adrenal suppression in children include linear growth retardation, delayed weight gain, low plasma cortisol levels, and absence of response to ACTH stimulation.

clinical pharmacology

Topical corticosteroids share anti-inflammatory, anti-pruritic and vasoconstrictive actions.

The mechanism of anti-inflammatory activity of the topical corticosteroids is unclear. Various laboratory methods, including vasoconstrictor assays, are used to compare and predict potencies and/or clinical efficacies of the topical corticosteroids. There is some evidence to suggest that a recognizable correlation exists between vasoconstrictor potency and therapeutic efficacy in man.

Pharmacokinetics

The extent of percutaneous absorption of topical corticosteroids is determined by many factors including the vehicle, the integrity of the epidermal barrier, and the use of occlusive dressings.

Topical corticosteroids can be absorbed from normal intact skin. Inflammation and/or other disease processes in the skin increase percutaneous absorption. Occlusive dressings substantially increase the percutaneous absorption of topical corticosteroids. Thus, occlusive dressings may be a valuable therapeutic adjunct for treatment of resistant dermatoses. (See *DOSAGE AND ADMINISTRATION*.)

Once absorbed through the skin, topical corticosteroids are handled through pharmacokinetic pathways similar to systemically administered corticosteroids. Corticosteroids are bound to plasma proteins in varying degrees. Corticosteroids are metabolized primarily in the liver and are then excreted by the kidneys. Some of the topical corticosteroids and their metabolites are also excreted into the bile.

indications and usage

SYNALAR® (fluocinolone acetonide) creams are indicated for the relief of the inflammatory and pruritic manifestations of corticosteroid-responsive dermatoses.

contraindications

Topical corticosteroids are contraindicated in those patients with a history of hypersensitivity to any of the components of the preparation.

precautions

General

Systemic absorption of topical corticosteroids has produced reversible hypothalamic-pituitary-adrenal (HPA) axis suppression, manifestations of Cushing's syndrome, hyperglycemia, and glucosuria in some patients.

Conditions which augment systemic absorption include the application of the more potent steroids, use over large surface areas, prolonged use, and the addition of occlusive dressings.

Therefore, patients receiving a large dose of a potent topical steroid applied to a large surface area or under an occlusive dressing should be evaluated periodically for evidence of HPA axis suppression by using the urinary free cortisol and ACTH stimulation tests. If HPA axis suppression is noted, an attempt should be made to withdraw the drug, to reduce the frequency of application, or to substitute a less potent steroid.

Recovery of HPA axis function is generally prompt and complete upon discontinuation of the drug. Infrequently, signs and symptoms of steroid withdrawal may occur, requiring supplemental systemic corticosteroids.

Children may absorb proportionally larger amounts of topical corticosteroids and thus be more susceptible to systemic toxicity. (See *PRECAUTIONS—Pediatric Use*.)

If irritation develops, topical corticosteroids should be discontinued and appropriate therapy instituted.

As with any topical corticosteroid product, prolonged use may produce atrophy of the skin and subcutaneous tissues. When used on intertriginous or flexor area, or on the face, this may occur even with short term use.

In the presence of dermatological infections, the use of an appropriate antifungal or antibacterial agent should be instituted. If a favorable response does not occur promptly, the corticosteroid should be discontinued until the infection has been adequately controlled.

Information for the Patient

Patients using topical corticosteroids should receive the following information and instructions:

1. This medication is to be used as directed by the physician. It is for external use only. Avoid contact with the eyes.
2. Patients should be advised not to use this medication for any disorder other than for which it was prescribed.

Manifestations of intracranial hypertension include bulging fontanelles, headaches, and bilateral papilledema.

Administration of topical corticosteroids to children should be limited to the least amount compatible with an effective therapeutic regimen. Chronic corticosteroid therapy may interfere with the growth and development of children.

adverse reactions

The following local adverse reactions are reported infrequently with topical corticosteroids, but may occur more frequently with the use of occlusive dressings. These reactions are listed in an approximate decreasing order of occurrence:

Burning	Hypertrichosis
Itching	Acneiform eruptions
Irritation	Hypopigmentation
Dryness	Perioral dermatitis
Folliculitis	Allergic contact dermatitis
Maceration of the skin	
Secondary infection	
Skin atrophy	
Striae	
Miliaria	

overdosage

Topically applied corticosteroids can be absorbed in sufficient amounts to produce systemic effects. (See *PRECAUTIONS*.)

dosage and administration

SYNALAR® (fluocinolone acetonide) creams are generally applied to the affected area as a thin film from two to four times daily depending on the severity of the condition. In hairy sites, the hair should be parted to allow direct contact with the lesion.

Occlusive dressing may be used for the management of psoriasis or recalcitrant conditions. Some plastic films may be flammable and due care should be exercised in their use. Similarly, caution should be employed when such films are used on children or left in their proximity, to avoid the possibility of accidental suffocation.

If an infection develops, the use of occlusive dressings should be discontinued and appropriate antimicrobial therapy instituted.

how supplied

SYNALAR® (fluocinolone acetonide) cream 0.025%

15 g Tube	—**NDC**	0033-2501-13
30 g Tube	—**NDC**	0033-2501-14
60 g Tube	—**NDC**	0033-2501-17
425 g Jar	—**NDC**	0033-2501-23

SYNALAR® (fluocinolone acetonide) cream 0.01%

15 g Tube	—**NDC**	0033-2502-13
30 g Tube	—**NDC**	0033-2502-14
60 g Tube	—**NDC**	0033-2502-17
425 g Jar	—**NDC**	0033-2502-23

Store tubes at room temperature; avoid freezing and excessive heat, above 40℃ (104°F).

Store jars at controlled room temperature, 15°–30°C (59°–86°F).

CAUTION: Federal law prohibits dispensing without prescription.

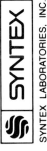

SYNTEX LABORATORIES, INC.
PALO ALTO, CA 94304

Revised OCTOBER 1989
© SYNTEX LABORATORIES, INC.

02-2502-14-00

LIDEX®

Products 0.05%
(fluocinonide)

Description LIDEX® (fluocinonide) products are intended for topical administration. Their active component is the corticosteroid fluocinonide, which is the 21-acetate ester of fluocinolone acetonide and has the chemical name pregna-1, 4-diene-3, 20-dione, 21-(acetyloxy)-6, 9-difluoro-11-hydroxy-16, 17-[(1-methylethylidene) bis (oxy)]-, (6α, 11β, 16α)-.

LIDEX cream 0.05% contains fluocinonide 0.5 mg/g in FAPG® cream, a specially formulated cream base consisting of citric acid, 1,2,6-hexanetriol, polyethylene glycol 8000, propylene glycol and stearyl alcohol. This white cream vehicle is greaseless, non-staining, anhydrous and completely water miscible. The base provides emollient and hydrophilic properties. In this formulation, the active ingredient is totally in solution.

LIDEX ointment 0.05% contains fluocinonide 0.5 mg/g in a specially formulated ointment base consisting of glyceryl monostearate, white petrolatum, propylene carbonate, propylene glycol and white wax. It provides the occlusive and emollient effects desirable in an ointment. In this formulation, the active ingredient is totally in solution.

LIDEX-E cream 0.05% contains fluocinonide 0.5 mg/g in a water-washable aqueous emollient base of cetyl alcohol, citric acid, mineral oil, polysorbate 60, propylene glycol, sorbitan monostearate, stearyl alcohol and water (purified).

LIDEX topical solution 0.05% contains fluocinonide 0.5 mg/mL in a solution of alcohol (35%), citric acid, disopropyl adipate and propylene glycol. In this formulation, the active ingredient is totally in solution.

LIDEX gel 0.05% contains fluocinonide 0.5 mg/mL in a specially formulated gel base consisting of carbomer 940, edetate disodium, propyl gallate, propylene glycol, sodium hydroxide and/or hydrochloric acid (to adjust pH) and water (purified). This clear, colorless thixotropic vehicle is greaseless, non-staining and completely water miscible. In this formulation, the active ingredient is totally in solution.

Clinical Pharmacology Topical corticosteroids share anti-inflammatory, antipruritic and vasoconstrictive actions.

The mechanism of anti-inflammatory activity of the topical corticosteroids is unclear. Various laboratory methods, including vasoconstrictor assays, are used to compare and predict potencies and/or clinical efficacies of the topical corticosteroids. There is some evidence to suggest that a recognizable correlation exists between vasoconstrictor potency and therapeutic efficacy in man.

Pharmacokinetics The extent of percutaneous absorption of topical corticosteroids is determined by many factors including the vehicle, the integrity of the epidermal barrier and the use of occlusive dressings. A significantly greater amount of fluocinonide is absorbed from the solution than from the cream or gel formulations.

Topical corticosteroids can be absorbed from normal intact skin. Inflammation and/or other disease processes in the skin increase percutaneous absorption. Occlusive dressings substantially increase the percutaneous absorption of topical corticosteroids. Thus, occlusive dressings may be a valuable therapeutic adjunct for treatment of resistant dermatoses. (See DOSAGE AND ADMINISTRATION.)

Once absorbed through the skin, topical corticosteroids are handled through pharmacokinetic pathways similar to systemically administered corticosteroids. Corticosteroids are bound to plasma proteins in varying degrees. Corticosteroids are metabolized primarily in the liver and are then excreted by the kidneys. Some of the topical corticosteroids and their metabolites are also excreted into the bile.

Indications and Usage These products are indicated for the relief of the inflammatory and pruritic manifestations of corticosteroid-responsive dermatoses.

Contraindications Topical corticosteroids are contraindicated in those patients with a history of hypersensitivity to any of the components of the preparation.

Precautions General Systemic absorption of topical corticosteroids has produced reversible hypothalamic-pituitary-adrenal (HPA) axis suppression, manifestations of Cushing's syndrome, hyperglycemia, and glucosuria in some patients.

Conditions which augment systemic absorption include the application of the more potent steroids, use over large surface areas, prolonged use, the addition of occlusive dressings, and dosage form.

Therefore, patients receiving a large dose of a potent topical steroid applied to a large surface area or under an occlusive dressing should be evaluated periodically for evidence of HPA axis suppression by using the urinary free cortisol and ACTH stimulation tests. If HPA axis suppression is noted, an attempt should be made to withdraw the drug, to reduce the frequency of application, or to substitute a less potent steroid.

Recovery of HPA axis function is generally prompt and complete upon discontinuation of the drug. Infrequently, signs and symptoms of steroid withdrawal may occur, requiring supplemental systemic corticosteroids.

1. This medication is to be used as directed by the physician. It is for external use only. Avoid contact with the eyes. If there is contact with the eyes and severe irritation occurs, immediately flush the eyes with a large volume of water.

2. Patients should be advised not to use this medication for any disorder other than that for which it was prescribed.

3. The treated skin area should not be bandaged or otherwise covered or wrapped as to be occlusive unless directed by the physician.

4. Patients should report any signs of local adverse reactions especially under occlusive dressing.

5. Parents of pediatric patients should be advised not to use tight-fitting diapers or plastic pants on a child being treated in the diaper area, as these garments may constitute occlusive dressings.

Laboratory Tests The following tests may be helpful in evaluating the HPA axis suppression:
Urinary free cortisol test
ACTH stimulation test

Carcinogenesis, Mutagenesis, and Impairment of Fertility Long-term animal studies have not been performed to evaluate the carcinogenic potential or the effect on fertility of topical corticosteroids.

Studies to determine mutagenicity with prednisolone and hydrocortisone have revealed negative results.

Pregnancy Category C Corticosteroids are generally teratogenic in laboratory animals when administered systemically at relatively low dosage levels. The more potent corticosteroids have been shown to be teratogenic after dermal application in laboratory animals. There are no adequate and well-controlled studies in pregnant women on teratogenic effects from topically applied corticosteroids. Therefore, topical corticosteroids should be used during pregnancy only if the potential benefit justifies the potential risk to the fetus. Drugs of this class should not be used extensively on pregnant patients, in large amounts, or for prolonged periods of time.

Nursing Mothers It is not known whether topical administration of corticosteroids could result in sufficient systemic absorption to produce detectable quantities in breast milk. Systemically administered corticosteroids are secreted into breast milk in quantities not likely to have a deleterious effect on the infant. Nevertheless, caution should be exercised when topical corticosteroids are administered to a nursing woman.

Pediatric Use Pediatric patients may demonstrate greater susceptibility to topical corticosteroid-induced HPA axis suppression and Cushing's syndrome than mature patients because of a larger skin surface area to body weight ratio.

Hypothalamic-pituitary-adrenal (HPA) axis suppression, Cushing's syndrome, and intracranial hypertension have been reported in children receiving topical corticosteroids. Manifestations of adrenal suppression in children include linear growth retardation, delayed weight gain, low plasma cortisol levels, and absence of response to ACTH stimulation. Manifestations of intracranial hypertension include bulging fontanelles, headaches, and bilateral papilledema.

Administration of topical corticosteroids in children should be limited to the least amount compatible with an effective therapeutic regimen. Chronic corticosteroid therapy may interfere with the growth and development of children.

Adverse Reactions The following local adverse reactions are reported infrequently with topical corticosteroids, but may occur more frequently with the use of occlusive dressings. These reactions are listed in an approximate decreasing order of occurrence: burning, itching, irritation, dryness, folliculitis, hypertrichosis, acneiform eruptions, hypopigmentation, perioral dermatitis, allergic contact dermatitis, maceration of the skin, secondary infection, skin atrophy, striae, miliaria.

Overdosage Topically applied corticosteroids can be absorbed in sufficient amounts to produce systemic effects. (See PRECAUTIONS.)

Dosage and Administration These products are generally applied to the affected area as a thin film from two to four times daily depending on the severity of the condition.

Occlusive dressings may be used for the management of psoriasis or recalcitrant conditions.

If an infection develops, the use of occlusive dressings should be discontinued and appropriate antimicrobial therapy instituted.

How Supplied LIDEX® (fluocinonide) cream 0.05%: 15 g Tube–NDC 0033-2511-13; 30 g Tube–NDC 0033-2511-14; 60 g Tube–NDC 0033-2511-17; 120 g Tube–NDC 0033-2511-22. Store at room temperature. Avoid excessive heat, above 40°C (104°F).

LIDEX® (fluocinonide) ointment 0.05%: 15 g Tube–NDC 0033-2514-13; 30 g Tube–NDC 0033-2514-14; 60 g Tube–NDC 0033-2514-17; 120 g Tube–NDC 0033-2514-22. Store at room temperature. Avoid temperature above 30°C (86°F).

LIDEX-E® (fluocinonide) cream 0.05%: 15 g Tube–NDC 0033-2513-13; 30 g Tube–NDC 0033-2513-14; 60 g Tube–NDC 0033-2513-17; 120 g Tube–NDC 0033-2513-22. Store at room temperature. Avoid excessive heat, above 40°C (104°F).

LIDEX® (fluocinonide) topical solution 0.05%: plastic squeeze bottles: 20 cc. NDC 0033-2517-44; 60 cc. NDC 0033-2517-46. Store at room temperature. Avoid excessive heat, above 40°C (104°F).

Children may absorb proportionally larger amounts of topical corticosteroids and thus be more susceptible to systemic toxicity. (See PRECAUTIONS–Pediatric Use.)

Not for ophthalmic use. Severe irritation is possible if fluocinonide contacts the eye. If that should occur, immediate flushing of the eye with a large volume of water is recommended.

If irritation develops, topical corticosteroids should be discontinued and appropriate therapy instituted.

As with any topical corticosteroid product, prolonged use may produce atrophy of the skin and subcutaneous tissues. When used on intertriginous or flexor area, or on the face, this may occur even with short-term use.

In the presence of dermatological infections, the use of an appropriate antifungal or antibacterial agent should be instituted. If a favorable response does not occur promptly, the corticosteroid should be discontinued until the infection has been adequately controlled.

Information for the Patient Patients using topical corticosteroids should receive the following information and instructions:

LIDEX® (fluocinonide) gel 0.05%: 15 g Tube–NDC 0033-2507-13; 30 g Tube–NDC 0033-2507-14; 60 g Tube–NDC 0033-2507-17; 120 g Tube–NDC 0033-2507-22. Store at controlled room temperature, 15–30°C (59–86°F).

CAUTION: Federal law prohibits dispensing without prescription.

August 1990

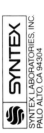

SYNTEX LABORATORIES, INC.
PALO ALTO, CA 94304

NASALIDE®
(flunisolide)
Nasal Solution 0.025%
For Nasal Use Only

DESCRIPTION

NASALIDE® (flunisolide) nasal solution is intended for administration as a spray to the nasal mucosa. Flunisolide, the active component of NASALIDE nasal solution, is an anti-inflammatory steroid with the chemical name: 6α-fluoro-11β,16α,17,21-tetrahydroxypregna-1,4-diene-3,20-dione cyclic 16,17-acetal with acetone (USAN). It has the following chemical structure:

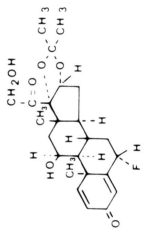

Flunisolide is a white to creamy white crystalline powder with a molecular weight of 434.49. It is soluble in acetone, sparingly soluble in chloroform, slightly soluble in methanol, and practically insoluble in water. It has a melting point of about 245°C.

Each 25 mL spray bottle contains flunisolide 6.25 mg (0.25 mg/mL) in a solution of propylene glycol, polyethylene glycol 3350, citric acid, sodium citrate, butylated hydroxyanisole, edetate disodium, benzalkonium chloride, and purified water, with NaOH and/or HCl added to adjust the pH to approximately 5.3. It contains no fluorocarbons.

After priming the delivery system for NASALIDE, each actuation of the unit delivers a metered droplet spray containing approximately 25 mcg of flunisolide. The size of the droplets produced by the unit is in excess of 8 microns to facilitate deposition on the nasal mucosa. The contents of one nasal spray bottle deliver at least 200 sprays.

CLINICAL PHARMACOLOGY

NASALIDE® (flunisolide) has demonstrated potent glucocorticoid and weak mineralocorticoid activity in classical animal test systems. As a glucocorticoid it is several hundred times more potent than the cortisol standard. Clinical studies with flunisolide have shown therapeutic activity on nasal mucous membranes with minimal evidence of systemic activity at the recommended doses.

A study in approximately 100 patients which compared the recommended dose of flunisolide nasal solution with an oral dose providing equivalent systemic amounts of flunisolide has shown that the clinical effectiveness of NASALIDE, when used topically as recommended, is due to its direct local effect and not to an indirect effect through systemic absorption.

Following administration of flunisolide to man, approximately half of the administered dose is recovered in the urine and half in the stool; 65-70% of the dose recovered in urine is the primary metabolite, which has undergone loss of the 6α fluorine and addition of a 6β hydroxy group. Flunisolide is well absorbed but is rapidly converted by the liver to the much less active primary metabolite and to glucuronate and/or sulfate conjugates. Because of first-pass liver metabolism, only 20% of the flunisolide reaches the systemic circulation when it is given orally whereas 50% of the flunisolide administered intranasally reaches the systemic circulation unmetabolized. The plasma half-life of flunisolide is 1-2 hours.

The effects of flunisolide on hypothalamic-pituitary-adrenal (HPA) axis function have been studied in adult volunteers. NASALIDE was administered intranasally as a spray in total doses over 7 times the recommended dose (2200 mcg, equivalent to 88 sprays/day) in 2 subjects for 4 days, about 3 times the recommended dose (800 mcg, equivalent to 32 sprays/day) in 4 subjects for 4 days, and over twice the recommended dose (700 mcg, equivalent to 28 sprays/day) in 6 subjects for 10 days. Early morning plasma cortisol concentrations and 24-hour urinary 17-ketogenic steroids were measured daily. There was evidence of decreased endogenous cortisol production at all three doses.

In controlled studies, NASALIDE was found to be effective in reducing symptoms of stuffy nose, runny nose and sneezing in most patients. These controlled clinical studies have been conducted in 488 adult patients at doses ranging from 8 to 16 sprays (200-400 mcg) per day and 127 children at doses ranging from 6 to 8 sprays (150-200 mcg) per day for periods as long as 3 months. In 170 patients who had cortisol levels evaluated at baseline and after 3 months or more of flunisolide treatment, there was no unequivocal flunisolide-related depression of plasma cortisol levels.

The mechanisms responsible for the anti-inflammatory action of corticosteroids and for the activity of the aerosolized drug on the nasal mucosa are unknown.

INDICATIONS

NASALIDE® (flunisolide) is indicated for the topical treatment of the symptoms of seasonal or perennial rhinitis when effectiveness of or tolerance to conventional treatment is unsatisfactory.

Clinical studies have shown that improvement is based on a local effect rather than systemic absorption, and is usually apparent within a few days after starting NASALIDE. However, symptomatic relief may not occur in some patients for as long as two weeks. Although systemic effects are minimal at recommended doses, NASALIDE should not be continued beyond 3 weeks in the absence of significant symptomatic improvement.

NASALIDE should not be used in the presence of untreated localized infection involving nasal mucosa.

CONTRAINDICATIONS

Hypersensitivity to any of the ingredients.

WARNINGS

The replacement of a systemic corticosteroid with a topical corticoid can be accompanied by signs of adrenal insufficiency, and in addition some patients may experience symptoms of withdrawal, e.g., joint and/or muscular pain, lassitude and depression. Patients previously treated for prolonged periods with systemic corticosteroids and transferred to NASALIDE® (flunisolide) should be carefully monitored to avoid acute adrenal insufficiency in response to stress.

When transferred to NASALIDE, careful attention must be given to patients previously treated for prolonged periods with systemic corticosteroids. This is particularly important in those patients who have associated asthma or other clinical conditions, where too rapid a decrease in systemic corticosteroids may cause a severe exacerbation of their symptoms.

The use of NASALIDE with alternate-day prednisone systemic treatment could increase the likelihood of HPA suppression compared to a therapeutic dose of either one alone. Therefore, NASALIDE treatment should be used with caution in patients already on alternate-day prednisone regimens for any disease.

PRECAUTIONS

General: In clinical studies with flunisolide administered intranasally, the development of localized infections of the nose and pharynx with *Candida albicans* has occurred only rarely. When such an infection develops it may require treatment with appropriate local therapy or discontinuance of treatment with NASALIDE® (flunisolide).

Flunisolide is absorbed into the circulation. Use of excessive doses of NASALIDE may suppress hypothalamic-pituitary-adrenal function.

Flunisolide should be used with caution, if at all in patients with active or quiescent tuberculosis infections of the respiratory tract or in untreated fungal, bacterial or systemic viral infections or ocular herpes simplex.

Because of the inhibitory effect of corticosteroids on wound healing, in patients who have experienced recent nasal septal ulcers, recurrent epistaxis, nasal surgery or trauma, a nasal corticosteroid should be used with caution until healing has occurred.

Although systemic effects have been minimal with recommended doses, this potential increases with excessive dosages. Therefore, larger than recommended doses should be avoided.

Information for Patients: Patients should use NASALIDE at regular intervals since its effectiveness depends on its regular use. The patient should take the medication as directed. It is not acutely effective and the prescribed dosage should not be increased. Instead, nasal vasoconstrictors or oral antihistamines may be needed until the effects of NASALIDE are fully manifested. One to two weeks may pass before full relief is obtained. The patient should contact the physician if symptoms do not improve, or if the condition worsens, or if sneezing or nasal irritation occurs.

For the proper use of this unit and to attain maximum improvement, the patient should read and follow the accompanying Patient Instructions carefully.

Carcinogenesis: Long-term studies were conducted in mice and rats using oral administration to evaluate the carcinogenic potential of the drug. There was an increase in the incidence of pulmonary adenomas in mice, but not in rats.

Female rats receiving the highest oral dose had an increased incidence of mammary adenocarcinoma compared to control rats. An increased incidence of this tumor type has been reported for other corticosteroids.

Impairment of fertility: Female rats receiving high doses of flunisolide (200 mcg/kg/day) showed some evidence of impaired fertility. Reproductive performance in the low (8 mcg/kg/day) and mid-dose (40 mcg/kg/day) groups was comparable to controls.

Pregnancy: Teratogenic effects: Pregnancy Category C. As with other corticosteroids, flunisolide has been shown to be teratogenic in rabbits and rats at doses of 40 and 200 mcg/kg/day respectively. It was also fetotoxic in these animal reproductive studies. There are no adequate and well-controlled studies in pregnant women. Flunisolide should be used during pregnancy only if the potential benefit justifies the potential risk to the fetus.

Nursing Mothers: It is not known whether this drug is excreted in human milk. Because other corticosteroids are excreted in human milk, caution should be exercised when flunisolide is administered to nursing women.

ADVERSE REACTIONS

Adverse reactions reported in controlled clinical trials and long-term open studies in 595 patients treated with NASALIDE are described below. Of these patients, 409 were treated for 3 months or longer, 323 for 6 months or longer, 259 for 1 year or longer, and 91 for 2 years or longer.

In general, side effects elicited in the clinical studies have been primarily associated with the nasal mucous membranes. The most frequent complaints were those of mild transient nasal burning and stinging, which were reported in approximately 45% of the patients treated with NASALIDE in placebo-controlled and long-term studies. These complaints do not usually interfere with treatment; in only 3% of patients was it necessary to decrease dosage or stop treatment because of these symptoms. Approximately the same incidence of mild transient nasal burning and stinging was reported in patients on placebo as was reported in patients treated with NASALIDE in controlled studies, implying that these complaints may be related to the vehicle or the delivery system. The incidence of complaints of nasal burning and stinging decreased with increasing duration of treatment.

Other side effects reported at a frequency of 5% or less were: nasal congestion, sneezing, epistaxis and/or bloody mucus, nasal irritation, watery eyes, sore throat, nausea and/or vomiting, headaches and loss of sense of smell and taste. As is the case with other nasally inhaled corticosteroids, nasal septal perforations have been observed in rare instances.

Systemic corticosteroid side effects were not reported during the controlled clinical trials. If recommended doses are exceeded, or if individuals are particularly sensitive, symptoms of hypercorticism, i.e., Cushing's syndrome, could occur.

OVERDOSAGE

I.V. flunisolide in animals at doses up to 4 mg/kg showed no effect. One spray bottle contains 6.25 mg of NASALIDE; therefore acute overdosage is unlikely.

DOSAGE AND ADMINISTRATION

The therapeutic effects of corticosteroids, unlike those of decongestants, are not immediate. This should be explained to the patient in advance in order to ensure cooperation and continuation of treatment with the prescribed dosage regimen. Full therapeutic benefit requires regular use, and is usually evident within a few days. However, a longer period of therapy may be required for some patients to achieve maximum benefit (up to 3 weeks). If no improvement is evident by that time, NASALIDE® (flunisolide) should not be continued.

Patients with blocked nasal passages should be encouraged to use a decongestant just before NASALIDE administration to ensure adequate penetration of the spray. Patients should also be advised to clear their nasal passages of secretions prior to use.

Adults: The recommended starting dose of NASALIDE is 2 sprays (50 mcg) in each nostril 2 times a day (total dose 200 mcg/day). If needed, this dose may be increased to 2 sprays in each nostril 3 times a day (total dose 300 mcg/day).

Children 6 to 14 years: The recommended starting dose of NASALIDE is one spray (25 mcg) in each nostril 3 times a day or two sprays (50 mcg) in each nostril 2 times a day (total dose 150-200 mcg/day). NASALIDE is not recommended for use in children less than 6 years of age as safety and efficacy studies, including possible adverse effects on growth, have not been conducted.

Maximum total daily doses should not exceed 8 sprays in each nostril for adults (total dose 400 mcg/day) and 4 sprays in each nostril for children under 14 years of age (total dose 200 mcg/day). Since there is no evidence that exceeding the maximum recommended dosage is more effective and increased systemic absorption would occur, higher doses should be avoided.

After the desired clinical effect is obtained, the maintenance dose should be reduced to the smallest amount necessary to control the symptoms. Approximately 15% of patients with perennial rhinitis may be maintained on as little as 1 spray in each nostril per day.

HOW SUPPLIED

Each 25 mL NASALIDE® (flunisolide) nasal solution spray bottle (NDC 0033-2906-40) (NSN 6505-01-132-9979) contains 6.25 mg (0.25 mg/mL) of flunisolide and is supplied in a nasal pump dispenser with dust cover and with a patient leaflet of instructions.

Store at controlled room temperature, 15°-30°C (59°-86°F).

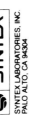 SYNTEX

SYNTEX LABORATORIES, INC.
PALO ALTO, CA 94304

02-2906-42-00

© Revised July 1988

TORADOL® IM
(ketorolac
tromethamine)

DESCRIPTION

TORADOL® (ketorolac tromethamine) is a member of the pyrrolo-pyrrole group of nonsteroidal anti-inflammatory drugs (NSAIDs). The chemical name for ketorolac tromethamine is (±)-5-benzoyl-2,3-dihydro-1H-pyrrolizine-1-carboxylic acid,2-amino-2-(hydroxymethyl)-1,3-propanediol and it has the following structure:

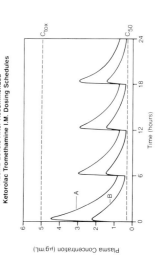

Plasma Levels After Recommended
Ketorolac Tromethamine I.M. Dosing Schedules

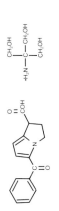

A = Ketorolac tromethamine 60 mg followed by 30 mg doses (Q 6 hr)
B = Ketorolac tromethamine 30 mg followed by 15 mg doses (Q 6 hr)
C_{tox} = Estimated concentration above which side effects are frequent
C_{50} = Estimated concentration required to obtain 50% decreases in pain intensity scores in dental surgery pain

Ketorolac tromethamine is soluble in water, has a pKa of 3.54 and an n-octanol/water partition coefficient of 0.26. The molecular weight of ketorolac tromethamine is 376.41.

TORADOL Injection is available for intramuscular (IM) administration as: 15 mg in 1 mL (1.5%), 30 mg in 1 mL (3%), or 60 mg in 2 mL (3%) of ketorolac tromethamine in sterile solution. The 15 mg/mL solution contains 10% (w.v) alcohol. USP. and 6.68 mg of sodium chloride in sterile water. The 30 mg/mL solution contains 10% (w.v) alcohol. USP. and 4.35 mg sodium chloride in sterile water. The pH is adjusted with sodium hydroxide or hydrochloric acid. The sterile solutions are clear and slightly yellow in color.

CLINICAL PHARMACOLOGY

Pharmacodynamics

TORADOL is a nonsteroidal anti-inflammatory drug (NSAID) that exhibits analgesic, anti-inflammatory, and antipyretic activity.

TORADOL inhibits synthesis of prostaglandins and may be considered a peripherally acting analgesic. Pain relief, following extraction of third impacted molars, is clinically evident when steady state plasma levels exceed 0.3 µg/mL, while side effects are frequent above concentrations of 5 µg/mL. Pain relief is often perceptible in about 10 minutes after TORADOL administration, but peak analgesia lags peak plasma levels by 45 to 90 minutes. Ketorolac tromethamine does not have any known effects on opiate receptors.

Table of Estimated Pharmacodynamic Parameters Following Intramuscular Doses of TORADOL

C_{50}est[1]	0.1 – 0.3 µg/mL
C_{tox}cest[2]	5 µg/mL

1 Estimated concentration required to obtain 50% decreases in pain intensity scores in dental surgery pain
2 Estimated concentration above which side effects are frequent

Pharmacokinetics (see Tables and Graph)

TORADOL is completely absorbed following intramuscular administration with mean peak plasma concentrations of 2.2 – 3.0 µg/mL occurring an average of 50 minutes after a single 30 mg dose. The terminal plasma half-life is 3.8 – 6.3 hours in young adults and 4.7 – 8.6 hours in elderly subjects (mean age 72). More than 99% of the ketorolac tromethamine in plasma is protein bound over a wide concentration range.

The pharmacokinetics of ketorolac tromethamine in man, following single or multiple intramuscular doses, are apparently linear, e.g. plasma levels are approximately proportional to dosage. Steady state plasma levels are achieved after dosing every 6 hours for one day. No changes in clearance occur with chronic dosing. Ketorolac, following intravenous and intramuscular administration, displays characteristics of a two-compartment model. In order to minimize the time delay in achieving adequate analgesic effect from the initial dose of a given regimen, a loading dose equal to twice the maintenance dose is recommended. This is based upon the pharmacokinetic principle that when the dosing interval is near the drug's half-life, the target steady-state plasma level is achieved faster if the first dose is twice the maintenance dose. Due to the two-compartment characteristics of TORADOL, the loading dose results in plasma levels during the first dosing interval that are higher than in subsequent intervals (see graph).

The primary route of excretion of ketorolac tromethamine and its metabolites (conjugates and a para-hydroxy metabolite) is in the urine (mean 91.4%) and the remainder (mean 6.1%) is excreted in the feces. In patients with serum creatinine values ranging from 1.9 to 5.0 mg/dl, the rate of ketorolac clearance was reduced to approximately half of normal.

Table of Approximate† Average Pharmacokinetic Parameters Following Intramuscular Doses of TORADOL

	15 mg	30 mg	60 mg
Bioavailability (extent)	100%	100%	100%
T_{max}[1] (min)	30 – 60	30 – 60	30 – 60
C_{max}[2] (µg/mL) [single dose]	1.0 – 1.4	2.2 – 3.0	4.0 – 4.5
C_{max}[2] (µg/mL) [steady state qid]	1.1 – 1.7	2.3 – 3.5	N/A*
C_{min}[3] (µg/mL) [steady state qid]	0.2 – 0.3	0.3 – 0.7	N/A
C_{ave}[4] (µg/mL) [steady state qid]	0.6 – 0.8	1.3 – 1.5	N/A
$Vd(\beta)$[5]		0.15 – 0.33 L/kg	

Dose metabolized	~50%
% Dose excreted in urine	91%
% Dose excreted in feces	6%
% Plasma protein binding	99%

* Not applicable because 60 mg is only recommended as a loading dose
1 Time-to-peak plasma concentration
2 Peak Plasma concentration
3 Trough plasma concentration
4 Average plasma concentration
5 Volume of distribution (calculated from mean clearance and terminal half-life)

† Derived from pharmacokinetic studies in 32 normal volunteers.

The Influence of Age, Liver and Kidney Function on the Clearance and Terminal Half-life of TORADOL[1]

Types of Subjects:	Total Clearance:[2] [in L/h/kg] mean (range)	Terminal Half-life: [in hours] mean (range)
Normal subjects (n = 8)	0.026 (0.017 – 0.046)	4.5 (3.8 – 5.0)
Patients with hepatic dysfunction (n = 7)	0.029 (0.013 – 0.066)	5.4 (2.2 – 6.9)
Patients with renal impairment (n = 10)	0.016 (0.007 – 0.043)	9.6 (3.2 – 15.7)
Healthy elderly subjects (n = 13)	0.019 (0.013 – 0.034)	7.0 (4.7 – 8.6)

1 Estimated from 30 mg single doses of ketorolac tromethamine
2 liters/hour/kilogram

Decreases in serum albumin, such as encountered in liver cirrhosis, would be expected to change ketorolac tromethamine clearance. However, in a study of 7 patients with liver cirrhosis, no correlation was found between serum albumin concentration and ketorolac tromethamine clearance.

Hemodynamics of anaesthetized patients were not altered by parenteral administration of TORADOL.

Ketorolac tromethamine poorly penetrates the blood-brain barrier (levels in the cerebrospinal fluid were found to be .002 times or less than those in plasma).

Clinical Studies

The analgesic efficacy of intramuscularly administered TORADOL was investigated in two post-operative pain models: general surgery (orthopedic, gynecologic and abdominal) and oral surgery (removal of impacted third molars). The studies were primarily double-blind, single-dose, parallel trial designs, in which TORADOL was compared to meperidine or morphine administered intramuscularly to patients with moderate to severe pain at baseline.

During the first hour, the onset of analgesic action was similar for TORADOL and the narcotics. TORADOL 30 or 90 mg intramuscularly, gave pain relief comparable to meperidine 100 mg or morphine 12 mg. TORADOL 10 mg was comparable to 50 mg of meperidine or 6 mg of morphine. The duration of analgesia was longer with all three doses of TORADOL. The percentage of patients who did not remedicate by 6 hours, i.e., by the end of the studies, was roughly 70%, 60% and 50% for TORADOL 90, 30 and 10 mg respectively, as compared to 30% and 20% for the high and low doses of the two narcotics.

In a multi-dose (10 doses), post-operative (general surgery) double-blind trial of TORADOL 30 mg versus morphine 6 and 12 mg, each drug given on an "as needed" basis, the overall analgesic effect of TORADOL 30 mg was in between that of morphine 6 and 12 mg. TORADOL 30 mg caused less drowsiness, nausea and vomiting than morphine 12 mg.

INDICATIONS AND USAGE

Intramuscular injection of TORADOL is indicated for the short-term management of pain (see "Clinical Studies" in CLINICAL PHARMACOLOGY).

TORADOL is not recommended for use as an obstetrical preoperative medication or for obstetrical analgesia because it has not been adequately studied for use in these circumstances and because of the known effects of drugs that inhibit prostaglandin biosynthesis on uterine contraction and fetal circulation.

TORADOL is not recommended for routine use with other nonsteroidal anti-inflammatory drugs (NSAIDs) because of the potential for additive side effects. TORADOL protein-binding is affected by aspirin (see PRECAUTIONS) but not by acetaminophen, ibuprofen, naproxen or piroxicam. Studies with other nonsteroidals have not been performed. TORADOL has been used concomitantly with morphine and meperidine without apparent adverse interactions.

CONTRAINDICATIONS

TORADOL should not be used in patients with previously demonstrated hypersensitivity to ketorolac tromethamine or in individuals with the complete or partial syndrome of nasal polyps, angioedema, and bronchospastic reactivity to aspirin or other nonsteroidal anti-inflammatory drugs (NSAIDs).

WARNINGS

Though TORADOL Injection is recommended for short-term use only, long-term administration of ketorolac tromethamine oral formulation has shown that this drug shares the risks that other nonsteroidal anti-inflammatory drugs (NSAIDs) pose to patients when taken chronically.

Risk of GI Ulcerations, Bleeding and Perforation with NSAID Treatment: Serious gastrointestinal toxicity, such as bleeding, ulceration, and perforation, can occur at any time, with or without warning symptoms, in patients treated chronically with NSAIDs. Although minor upper gastrointestinal problems, such as dyspepsia, are common, usually developing early in therapy, physicians should remain alert for ulceration and bleeding in patients treated chronically with NSAIDs, even in the absence of previous GI tract symptoms. In patients observed in clinical trials of such agents for several months to two years, symptomatic upper GI ulcers, gross bleeding or perforation appear to occur in approximately 1% of patients treated for 3-6 months, and in about 2-4% of patients treated for one year. Physicians should inform patients about the signs and/or symptoms of serious GI toxicity and what steps to take if they occur.

Studies to date have not identified any subset of patients not at risk of developing peptic ulceration and bleeding. Except for a prior history of serious GI events, and other risk factors known to be associated with peptic ulcer disease, such as alcoholism, smoking, etc., no risk factors (e.g., age, sex) have been associated with increased risk. Elderly or debilitated patients seem to tolerate ulceration or bleeding less well than other individuals, and most spontaneous reports of fatal GI events are in this population.

Studies to date are inconclusive concerning the relative risk of various nonsteroidal anti-inflammatory drugs (NSAIDs) in causing such reactions. High doses of any such agent probably carry a greater risk of these reactions, although controlled clinical trials showing this do not exist in most instances. In considering the use of relatively large doses (within the recommended dosage range), sufficient benefit should be anticipated to offset the potential increased risk of GI toxicity.

Because serious GI tract ulceration and bleeding can occur without warning symptoms, physicians should follow chronically treated patients for the signs and symptoms of ulceration and bleeding, and should inform the patients of the importance of this follow-up.

PRECAUTIONS

General Precautions

Impaired Renal or Hepatic Function: As with other nonsteroidal anti-inflammatory drugs (NSAIDs), TORADOL* should be used with caution in patients with impaired renal or hepatic function, or a history of kidney or liver disease. Studies to assess the pharmacokinetics of TORADOL in patients with active hepatitis or cholestasis have not been done.

Renal Effects: As with other nonsteroidal anti-inflammatory drugs, long-term administration of ketorolac tromethamine to animals resulted in renal papillary necrosis and other abnormal renal pathology. In humans, hematuria and proteinuria have been observed in long-term trials with oral ketorolac tromethamine treatment with a frequency and degree similar to the aspirin control group.

A second form of renal toxicity has been seen in patients with conditions leading to a reduction in blood volume and/or renal blood flow, where renal prostaglandins have a supportive role in the maintenance of renal perfusion. In these patients, administration of a nonsteroidal anti-inflammatory drug may cause a dose-dependent reduction in renal prostaglandin formation and may precipitate overt renal failure. Patients at greatest risk of this reaction are those with impaired renal function, heart failure, liver dysfunction, those taking diuretics and the elderly. Discontinuation of NSAID therapy is typically followed by recovery to the pretreatment state.

TORADOL and its metabolites are eliminated primarily by the kidneys which, in patients with reduced creatinine clearance, will result in diminished clearance of the drug (see CLINICAL PHARMACOLOGY). Therefore, TORADOL should be used with caution in patients with impaired renal function (see DOSAGE AND ADMINISTRATION section) and such patients should be followed closely. TORADOL has not been studied in patients with serum creatinine above 5.0 mg/dl, nor was it studied in patients on renal dialysis.

Fluid Retention and Edema: Fluid retention and edema have been reported with the use of NSAIDs; therefore, TORADOL should be used with caution in patients with cardiac decompensation, hypertension, or similar conditions.

Hepatic Effects: As with other nonsteroidal anti-inflammatory drugs (NSAIDs), borderline elevations of one or more liver tests may occur in up to 15% of patients. These abnormalities may progress, may remain essentially unchanged, or may disappear with continued therapy. The ALT (SGPT) test is probably the most sensitive indicator of liver injury. Meaningful (3 times the upper limit of normal) elevations of ALT or AST (SGOT) have been reported in controlled clinical trials (with the oral formulations of ketorolac tromethamine) in less than 1% of patients. A patient with symptoms and/or signs suggesting liver dysfunction, or in whom an abnormal liver test has occurred, should be evaluated for evidence of the development of a more severe hepatic reaction while on therapy with TORADOL. (See also Pharmacokinetics).

Hematologic Effects: TORADOL inhibits platelet aggregation and may prolong bleeding time. TORADOL does not affect platelet count, prothrombin time (PT) or partial thromboplastin time (PTT). Patients who have coagulation disorders or are receiving drug therapy that interferes with hemostasis should be carefully observed when TORADOL is administered. Unlike the prolonged effects from aspirin, the inhibition of platelet function by TORADOL disappears within 24 to 48 hours after the drug is discontinued. In controlled clinical studies, the incidence of clinically significant postoperative bleeding was 5/1170 (0.4%) compared to 1/570 (0.2%) in the control groups receiving opiates.

Drug Interactions

TORADOL is highly bound to human plasma protein (mean 99.2%), and binding is independent of concentration.

The in vitro binding of warfarin to plasma proteins is only slightly reduced by TORADOL (99.5% control vs 99.3% binding with TORADOL concentrations of 5 to 10 µg/mL). TORADOL does not alter digoxin protein binding.

In vitro studies indicated that at therapeutic concentrations of salicylate (300 µg/mL), the binding of TORADOL was reduced from approximately 99.2% to 97.5%, representing a potential two-fold increase in unbound TORADOL plasma levels; hence, TORADOL should be used with caution (or at a reduced dosage) in patients being treated with high dose salicylate regimens. Therapeutic concentrations of digoxin, warfarin, ibuprofen, naproxen, acetaminophen, phenytoin, tolbutamide and piroxicam did not alter TORADOL protein binding.

In a study of 12 healthy volunteers given TORADOL 10 mg orally for 6 days prior to co-administration of a single dose of warfarin 25 mg, no significant changes in pharmacokinetics or pharmacodynamics of warfarin were detected.

In another study of 12 healthy volunteers, co-administration of heparin 5000 U s.c. and TORADOL did not show any pharmacodynamic effects of the combination on template bleeding time or kaolin cephalin clotting time.

There is no evidence, in animal or human studies, that TORADOL induces or inhibits the hepatic enzymes capable of metabolizing itself or other drugs.

Lactation and Nursing

After a single oral administration of 10 mg of TORADOL to humans, the maximum milk concentration observed was 7.3 ng/mL and the maximum milk-to-plasma ratio was 0.037. After one day of dosing (qid), the maximum milk concentration was 7.9 ng/mL and the maximum milk-to-plasma ratio was 0.025. Caution should be exercised when TORADOL is administered to a nursing woman.

Pediatric Use

Safety and efficacy in children have not been established. Therefore, TORADOL is not recommended for use in children.

Use in the Elderly

Because ketorolac tromethamine is cleared somewhat more slowly by the elderly (see CLINICAL PHARMACOLOGY) who are also more sensitive to the renal effects of NSAIDs (see PRECAUTIONS Renal Effects), extra caution and reduced dosages (see DOSAGE AND ADMINISTRATION) should be used when treating the elderly with TORADOL.

ADVERSE REACTIONS

Adverse reactions rates from short-term use of NSAIDs are generally from 1/2 to 1/10 the rates associated with chronic usage. This is also true for TORADOL.

In studies of patients with chronic painful conditions treated for up to 1 year, the incidence of serious and nonserious ADRs, including GI tract ulceration and bleeding (yearly rate 1.2 to 5.4%), associated with 10 mg of ketorolac tromethamine orally, 1 to 4 times per day prn, was comparable to treatment with aspirin 650 mg on a similar prn schedule. Physicians using TORADOL should be alert for the usual complications of NSAID-treatment.

The adverse reactions listed below were reported to be probably related to TORADOL in clinical trials in which patients received up to 20 doses, in five days, of intramuscularly administered TORADOL 30 mg. Reactions are listed under body systems which are arranged alphabetically.

Incidence greater than 1%

Body as a whole: edema

Gastrointestinal: nausea*, dyspepsia*, gastrointestinal pain*, diarrhea

Nervous system: drowsiness*, dizziness, headache, sweating

Injection site pain was reported by 2% of patients in multidose studies (vs. 5% for morphine control group).

*Incidence of reported reaction between 3% and 9%. Those reactions occurring in less than 3% of the patients are unmarked.

Incidence 1% or less

Body as a whole: asthenia, myalgia

Cardiovascular: vasodilation, pallor

Dermatologic: pruritus, urticaria

Gastrointestinal: constipation, flatulence, gastrointestinal fullness, liver function abnormalities, melena, peptic ulcer, rectal bleeding, stomatitis, vomiting

Hemic and lymphatic: purpura

Nervous system: dry mouth, nervousness, paresthesia, abnormal thinking, depression, euphoria, excessive thirst, inability to concentrate, insomnia, stimulation, vertigo

Respiratory: dyspnea, asthma

Special senses: abnormal taste, abnormal vision

Urogenital: increased urinary frequency, oliguria

DRUG ABUSE AND PHYSICAL DEPENDENCE

TORADOL is not a narcotic agonist or antagonist. Subjects did not show any subjective symptoms or objective signs of drug withdrawal upon abrupt discontinuation of intravenous or intramuscular dosing. Patients receiving TORADOL orally for six months or longer have not developed tolerance to the drug and there is no pharmacologic basis to expect addiction. TORADOL did not exhibit activity in classical animal studies which are reasonable predictors of opiate analgesic action. In vitro, TORADOL does not bind to opiate receptors. These studies demonstrate that TORADOL does not have central opiate-like activity.

OVERDOSAGE

The absence of experience with acute overdosage precludes characterization of sequelae and assessment of antidotal efficacy at this time. At single oral doses greater than 100 mg/kg in rats, mice and monkeys, symptoms such as decreased activity, diarrhea, pallor, labored breathing, rales, and vomiting were observed.

DOSAGE AND ADMINISTRATION

TORADOL may be used on a regular schedule or prn ("as needed"), although current recommendations for pain management are to use analgesics on a regular schedule, rather than using them prn based on the return of pain. For the short-term management of pain (see CLINICAL PHARMACOLOGY for details of clinical trials), the recommended initial dose is 30 or 60 mg IM, as a loading dose, followed by half of the loading dose, e.g., 15 or 30 mg, every 6 hours as long as needed to control pain. The rationale for the recommended loading dose (LD) and the maintenance dosages (MD) is based upon pharmacokinetic and pharmacodynamic considerations (see CLINICAL PHARMACOLOGY): 60 mg LD/30 mg MD and 30 mg LD/15 mg MD above average plasma levels of 1.5 and 0.8 µg/mL respectively, which lie within the therapeutic range of 0.3 – 5 µg/mL. The recommended maximum total daily dose is 150 mg for the first day and 120 mg/day thereafter.

Inhibition of renal lithium clearance leading to an increase in plasma lithium concentration has been reported with some prostaglandin synthesis inhibiting drugs. The effect of TORADOL on plasma lithium levels has not been studied.

Concomitant administration of methotrexate and some NSAIDs has been reported to reduce the clearance of methotrexate, enhancing the toxicity of methotrexate. The effect of TORADOL on methotrexate clearance has not been studied.

Ketorolac tromethamine has been administered concurrently with morphine in several clinical trials of post-operative pain without evidence of adverse interactions.

Carcinogenesis, Mutagenesis, and Impairment of Fertility

An 18-month study in mice at oral doses of ketorolac tromethamine equal to the parenteral MRHD (Maximum Recommended Human Dose) and a 24-month study in rats at oral doses 2.5 times the parenteral MRHD, showed no evidence of tumorigenicity.

Ketorolac tromethamine was not mutagenic in tests performed with S. typhimurium, S. cerevisiae, or E. coli. Ketorolac did not cause chromosome breakage in the *in vivo* mouse micronucleus assay.

Impairment of fertility did not occur in male or female rats at oral doses of 9 mg/kg (4.5 times the parenteral MRHD) and 16 mg/kg (8 times the parenteral MRHD), respectively.

Pregnancy:

Pregnancy – Category B

Reproduction studies have been performed in rabbits, using daily oral doses equal to 3.6 mg/kg (1.8 times the parenteral Maximum Recommended Human Dose – MRHD) and, in rats, equal to 10 mg/kg (5 times the parenteral MRHD), respectively, and did not reveal evidence of harm to the fetus. Ketorolac tromethamine caused delayed parturition and dystocia in rats at oral doses higher than the parenteral MRHD, like other inhibitors of prostaglandin synthesis. There are, however, no adequate and well-controlled studies in pregnant women. Because animal reproduction studies are not always predictive of human response, this drug should be used during pregnancy only if clearly needed and no known safer alternatives are available.

Labor and Delivery

TORADOL is not recommended for use during labor and delivery (see INDICATIONS).

If prn management is elected, however, since the half-life of TORADOL is approximately – hours, an assessment of the size of a repeat dose can be based on the duration of pain relief from the previous dose. For exam ple, if pain returns within 3-5 hours the next dose could be increased by up to 50%. [Note: The recommended maximum total daily dose is 120 mg (150 mg on the first day). An alternative would be to use morphine or meperidine concomitantly (see INDICATIONS and DRUG INTERACTIONS). Alternatively, if pain does not return for 8 to 12 hours, the next dose could be decreased b as much as 50%, or the previous dose could be given every 8 to 12 hours.

The lower end of the recommended dosage range is recommended for patients under 5 kg (110 pounds), for patients over 65 years of age, and for patients with reduced renal function (see CLINICAL PHARMACOL Y and PRECAUTIONS).

HOW SUPPLIED

TORADOL® **IM** (ketorolac tromethamine) for single-dose intramuscular use is available in:

15 mg: 15 mg/mL, 1 mL Cartrix® syringe
(box of 10)
NDC #0033-2443-40

30 mg: 30 mg/mL, 1 mL Cartrix syringe
(box of 10)
NDC #0033-2434-40

60 mg: 30 mg/mL, 2 mL Cartrix syringe
(box of 10)
NDC #0033-2444-40

Store at controlled room temperature 15–30°C (59-86°F) with protection from light.

CAUTION: Federal law prohibits dispensing without prescription.

U.S. Patent No. 4,089,969 and others.

Mfd. for Syntex Laboratories, Inc.
Palo Alto, CA 94304
by Survival Technology, Inc.
Bethesda, MD 20814

02-2434-40-00

© Sy tex Laboratories, Inc. December 1989

SYNTEX

CARDENE®
(nicardipine hydrochloride)

Capsules

DESCRIPTION

CARDENE® capsules for oral administration each contain 20 mg or 30 mg of nicardipine hydrochloride. CARDENE is a calcium ion influx inhibitor (slow channel blocker or calcium channel blocker).

Nicardipine hydrochloride is a dihydropyridine structure with the IUPAC (International Union of Pure and Applied Chemistry) chemical name 2-(benzyl-methyl amino)ethyl methyl 1,4-dihydro-2,6-dimethyl-4-(*m*-nitrophenyl)-3,5-pyridinedicarboxylate monohydrochloride, and it has the following structure:

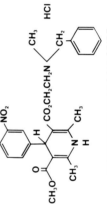

NICARDIPINE HYDROCHLORIDE

Nicardipine hydrochloride is a greenish-yellow, odorless, crystalline powder that melts at about 169°C. It is freely soluble in chloroform, methanol, and glacial acetic acid, sparingly soluble in anhydrous ethanol, slightly soluble in n-butanol, water, 0.01 M potassium dihydrogen phosphate, acetone, and dioxane, very slightly soluble in ethyl acetate, and practically insoluble in benzene, ether and hexane. It has a molecular weight of 515.99.

CARDENE is available in hard gelatin capsules containing 20 mg or 30 mg nicardipine hydrochloride with magnesium stearate and pregelatinized starch as the inactive ingredients. The 20 mg strength is provided in opaque white-white capsules made tamper evident by a brilliant blue gelatin band while the 30 mg capsules are opaque light blue-powder blue with a brilliant blue gelatin band. The colorants used in the 20 mg capsules are titanium dioxide, D&C Red #7 Calcium Lake and FD&C Blue #1 and the 30 mg capsules use titanium dioxide, FD&C Yellow #10 Aluminum Lake, D&C Red #7 Calcium Lake, and FD&C Blue #2.

CLINICAL PHARMACOLOGY

Mechanism of Action

CARDENE is a calcium entry blocker (slow channel blocker or calcium ion antagonist) which inhibits the transmembrane influx of calcium ions into cardiac muscle and smooth muscle without changing serum calcium concentrations. The contractile processes of cardiac muscle and vascular smooth muscle are dependent upon the movement of extracellular calcium ions into these cells through specific ion channels. The effects of CARDENE are more selective to vascular smooth muscle than cardiac muscle. In animal models, CARDENE produces relaxation of coronary vascular smooth muscle at drug levels which cause little or no negative inotropic effect.

Pharmacokinetics and Metabolism

CARDENE is completely absorbed following oral doses administered as capsules. Plasma levels are detectable as early as 20 minutes following an oral dose and maximal plasma levels are observed within 30 minutes to two hours (mean T_{max} = 1 hour). While CARDENE is completely absorbed, it is subject to saturable first pass metabolism and the systemic bioavailability is about 35% following a 30 mg oral dose at steady state.

When CARDENE was administered one (1) or three (3) hours after a high fat meal, the mean Cmax and mean AUC were lower (20% to 30%) than when CARDENE was given in fasting subjects. These decreases in plasma levels observed following a meal may be significant but the clinical trials establishing the efficacy and safety of CARDENE were done in patients without regard to the timing of meals. Thus the results of these trials reflect the effects of meal-induced variability.

The pharmacokinetics of CARDENE are nonlinear due to saturable hepatic first pass metabolism. Following oral administration, increasing doses result in a disproportionate increase in plasma levels. Steady state Cmax values following 20, 30, and 40 mg doses every 8 hours averaged 36, 88, and 133 ng/mL, respectively. Hence, increasing the dose from 20 to 30 mg every 8 hours more than doubled Cmax and increasing the dose from 20 to 40 mg every 8 hours increased Cmax more than 3-fold. A similar disproportionate increase in AUC with dose was observed. Considerable inter-subject variability in plasma levels was also observed.

Post-absorption kinetics of CARDENE are also non-linear, although there is a reproducible terminal plasma half-life that averaged 8.6 hours following 30 and 40 mg doses at steady state (TID). The terminal half-life represents the elimination of less than 5% of the absorbed drug (measured by plasma concentrations). Elimination over the first 8 hours after dosing is much faster with a half-life of 2-4 hours. Steady state plasma levels are achieved after 2 to 3 days of TID dosing (every 8 hours) and are 2-fold higher than after a single dose.

CARDENE is highly protein bound (>95%) in human plasma over a wide concentration range.

CARDENE is metabolized extensively by the liver; less than 1% of intact drug is detected in the urine. Following a radioactive oral dose in solution, 60% of the radioactivity was recovered in the urine and 35% in feces. Most of the dose (over 90%) was recovered within 48 hours of dosing. CARDENE does not induce its own metabolism and does not induce hepatic microsomal enzymes.

The steady-state pharmacokinetics of CARDENE in elderly hypertensive patients (>65 years) are similar to those obtained in young normal adults. After one week of CARDENE dosing at 20 mg three times a day, the Cmax, Tmax, AUC, terminal plasma half-life, and the extent of protein binding of CARDENE observed in healthy elderly hypertensive patients did not differ significantly from those observed in young normal volunteers.

CARDENE plasma levels were higher in patients with mild renal impairment (baseline serum creatinine concentration ranged from 1.2 to 5.5 mg/dl) than in normal subjects. After 30 mg CARDENE TID at steady state, Cmax and AUC were approximately 2-fold higher in these patients.

Because CARDENE is extensively metabolized by the liver, the plasma levels of the drug are influenced by changes in hepatic function. CARDENE plasma levels were higher in patients with severe liver disease (hepatic cirrhosis confirmed by liver biopsy or presence of endoscopically-confirmed esophageal varices) than in normal subjects. After 20 mg CARDENE BID at steady state, Cmax and AUC were 1.8 and 4-fold higher, and the terminal half-life was prolonged to 19 hours in these patients.

Hemodynamics

In man, CARDENE produces a significant decrease in systemic vascular resistance. The degree of vasodilation and the resultant hypotensive effects are more prominent in hypertensive patients. In hypertensive patients, nicardipine reduces the blood pressure at rest and during isometric and dynamic exercise. In normotensive patients, a small decrease of about 9 mmHg in systolic and 7 mmHg in diastolic blood pressure may accompany this fall in peripheral resistance. An increase in heart rate may occur in response to the vasodilation and decrease in blood pressure, and in a few patients this heart rate increase may be pronounced. In clinical studies mean heart rate at time of peak plasma levels was usually increased by 5-10 beats per minute compared to placebo, with the greater increases at higher doses, while there was no difference from placebo at the end of the dosing interval. Hemodynamic studies following intravenous dosing in patients with coronary artery disease and normal or moderately abnormal left ventricular function have shown significant increases in ejection fraction and cardiac output with no significant change, or a decrease in left ventricular end-diastolic pressure (LVEDP). Although there is evidence that CARDENE increases coronary blood flow, there is no evidence that this effect plays any role in its effectiveness in stable angina. In patients with coronary artery disease, intracoronary administration of nicardipine caused no direct myocardial depression. CARDENE does, however, have a negative inotropic effect in some patients with severe left ventricular dysfunction and could, in patients with very impaired function, lead to worsened failure.

"Coronary Steal", the detrimental redistribution of coronary blood flow in patients with coronary artery disease (diversion of blood from underperfused areas toward better perfused areas) has not been observed during nicardipine treatment. On the contrary, nicardipine has been shown to improve systolic shortening in normal and hypokinetic segments of myocardial muscle, and radio-nuclide angiography has confirmed that wall motion remained improved during an increase in oxygen demand. Nonetheless, occasional patients have developed increased angina upon receiving nicardipine. Whether this represents steal in those patients, or is the result of increased heart rate and decreased diastolic pressure, is not clear.

In patients with coronary artery disease nicardipine improves L.V. diastolic distensibility during the early filling phase, probably due to a faster rate of myocardial relaxation in previously underperfused areas. There is little or no effect on normal myocardium, suggesting the improvement is mainly by indirect mechanisms such as afterload reduction, and reduced ischemia. Nicardipine has no negative effect on myocardial relaxation at therapeutic doses. The clinical consequences of these properties are as yet undemonstrated.

Electrophysiologic Effects

In general, no detrimental effects on the cardiac conduction system were seen with the use of CARDENE.

CARDENE increased the heart rate when given intravenously during acute electrophysiologic studies, and prolonged the corrected QT interval to a minor degree. The sinus node recovery times and SA conduction times were not affected by the drug. The PA, AH, and HV intervals* and the functional and effective refractory periods of the atrium were not prolonged by CARDENE and the relative and effective refractory periods of the His-Purkinje system were slightly shortened after intravenous CARDENE.

*PA = conduction time from high to low right atrium, AH = conduction time from low right atrium to His bundle deflection, or AV nodal conduction time, HV = conduction time through the His bundle and the bundle branch-Purkinje system.

Renal Function

There is a transient increase in electrolyte excretion, including sodium. CARDENE does not cause generalized fluid retention, as measured by weight changes, although 7-8% of the patients experience pedal edema.

Effects in Angina Pectoris

In controlled clinical trials of up to 12 weeks duration in patients with chronic stable angina, CARDENE increased exercise tolerance and reduced nitroglycerin consumption and the frequency of anginal attacks. The antianginal efficacy of CARDENE (20-40 mg) has been demonstrated in four placebo-controlled studies involving 258 patients with chronic stable angina. In exercise tolerance testing, CARDENE significantly increased time to angina, total exercise duration and time to 1 mm ST segment depression. Included among these four studies was a dose-definition study in which dose-related improvements in exercise tolerance at one marginal (10 mg TID) dosing and two effective-control doses (20 and 30 mg TID) were seen at all doses of 10, 20 and 30 mg TID. Effectiveness at 10 mg TID was, however, different from placebo at peak blood levels. CARDENE has been demonstrated over long-term dosing. Blood pressure fell in patients with angina by about 10/8 mmHg at peak blood levels and was little different from placebo at trough blood levels.

Effects in Hypertension

CARDENE produced dose-related decreases in both systolic and diastolic blood pressure in clinical trials. The antihypertensive efficacy of CARDENE administered three times daily has been demonstrated in three placebo-controlled studies involving 517 patients with mild to moderate hypertension. The blood pressure responses in the three studies were statistically significant from placebo at peak (1 hour post-dosing) and trough (8 hours post-dosing), although it is apparent that well over half of the antihypertensive effect is lost by the end of the dosing interval. The results from placebo controlled studies of CARDENE given three times daily are shown in the following table:

Dose	Number of Patients	SYSTOLIC BP (mmHg) Mean Peak Response	Mean Trough Response	Trough/ Peak	Dose	Number of Patients	DIASTOLIC BP (mmHg) Mean Peak Response	Mean Trough Response	Trough/ Peak
20 mg	50 52	−10.3 −17.6	−4.9 −7.9	48% 45%	20 mg	50 52	−10.6 − 9.0	−4.6 −2.9	43% 32%
30 mg	45 44	−14.5 −14.6	−7.2 −7.5	50% 51%	30 mg	45 44	−12.8 −14.2	−4.9 −4.3	38% 30%
40 mg	50 38	−16.3 −15.9	−9.5 −6.0	58% 38%	40 mg	50 38	−15.4 −14.8	−5.9 −3.7	38% 25%

The responses are shown as differences from the concurrent placebo control group. The large changes between peak and trough effects were not accompanied by observed side effects at peak response times. In a study using 24 hour intra-arterial blood pressure monitoring, the circadian variation in blood pressure remained unaltered, but the systolic and diastolic blood pressures were reduced throughout the whole 24 hours.

When added to beta-blocker therapy, CARDENE further lowers both systolic and diastolic blood pressure.

INDICATIONS AND USAGE

I. Stable Angina

CARDENE is indicated for the management of patients with chronic stable angina (effort-associated angina). CARDENE may be used alone or in combination with beta-blockers.

II. Hypertension

CARDENE is indicated for the treatment of hypertension. CARDENE may be used alone or in combination with other antihypertensive drugs. In administering nicardipine it is important to be aware of the relatively large peak to trough differences in blood pressure effect. (See DOSAGE AND ADMINISTRATION.)

CONTRAINDICATIONS

CARDENE is contraindicated in patients with hypersensitivity to the drug.

Because part of the effect of CARDENE is secondary to reduced afterload, the drug is also contraindicated in patients with advanced aortic stenosis. Reduction of diastolic pressure in these patients may worsen rather than improve myocardial oxygen balance.

WARNINGS

Increased Angina

About 7% of patients in short term placebo-controlled angina trials have developed increased frequency, duration or severity of angina on starting CARDENE or at the time of dosage increases, compared with 4% of patients on placebo. Comparisons with beta-blockers also show a greater frequency of increased angina, 4% vs 1%. The mechanism of this effect has not been established. (See ADVERSE REACTIONS.)

Use in Patients with Congestive Heart Failure

Although preliminary hemodynamic studies in patients with congestive heart failure have shown that CARDENE reduced afterload without impairing myocardial contractility, it has a negative inotropic effect in vitro and in some patients. Caution should be exercised when using the drug in congestive heart failure patients, particularly in combination with a beta-blocker.

Beta-Blocker Withdrawal

CARDENE is not a beta-blocker and therefore gives no protection against the dangers of abrupt beta-blocker withdrawal; any such withdrawal should be by gradual reduction of the dose of beta-blocker, preferably over 8-10 days.

PRECAUTIONS

GENERAL

Blood Pressure: Because CARDENE decreases peripheral resistance, careful monitoring of blood pressure during the initial administration and titration of CARDENE is suggested. CARDENE, like other calcium channel blockers, may occasionally produce symptomatic hypotension. Caution is advised to avoid systemic hypotension when administering the drug to patients who have sustained an acute cerebral infarction or hemorrhage. Because of prominent effects at the time of peak blood levels, initial titration should be performed with measurements of blood pressure at peak effect (1-2 hours after dosing) and just before the next dose.

Use in patients with impaired hepatic function: Since the liver is the major site of biotransformation and since CARDENE is subject to first pass metabolism, the drug should be used with caution in patients having impaired liver function or reduced hepatic blood flow. Patients with severe liver disease developed elevated blood levels (4-fold increase in AUC) and prolonged half-life (19 hours) of CARDENE. (See DOSAGE AND ADMINISTRATION.)

Use in patients with impaired renal function: When CARDENE 20 mg or 30 mg TID was given to hypertensive patients with mild renal impairment, mean plasma concentrations, AUC, and Cmax were approximately 2-fold higher in renally impaired patients than in healthy controls. Doses in these patients must be adjusted. (See CLINICAL PHARMACOLOGY and DOSAGE AND ADMINISTRATION.)

DRUG INTERACTIONS

Beta-Blockers

In controlled clinical studies, adrenergic beta-receptor blockers have been frequently administered concomitantly with CARDENE. The combination is well tolerated.

Cimetidine

Cimetidine increases CARDENE plasma levels. Patients receiving the two drugs concomitantly should be carefully monitored.

Digoxin

Some calcium blockers may increase the concentration of digitalis preparations in the blood. CARDENE usually does not alter the plasma levels of digoxin, however, serum digoxin levels should be evaluated after concomitant therapy with CARDENE is initiated.

Maalox

Co-administration of Maalox TC had no effect on CARDENE absorption.

Fentanyl Anesthesia

Severe hypotension has been reported during fentanyl anesthesia with concomitant use of a beta-blocker and a calcium channel blocker. Even though such interactions were not seen during clinical studies with CARDENE, an increased volume of circulating fluids might be required if such an interaction were to occur.

Cyclosporine

Concomitant administration of nicardipine and cyclosporine results in elevated plasma cyclosporine levels. Plasma concentrations of cyclosporine should therefore be closely monitored, and its dosage reduced accordingly, in patients treated with nicardipine.

When therapeutic concentrations of *furosemide, propranolol, dipyridamole, warfarin, quinidine,* or *naproxen* were added to human plasma (*in vitro*), the plasma protein binding of CARDENE was not altered.

Carcinogenesis, Mutagenesis, Impairment of Fertility

Rats treated with nicardipine in the diet (at concentrations calculated to provide daily dosage levels of 5, 15 or 45 mg/kg/day) for two years showed a dose-dependent increase in thyroid hyperplasia and neoplasia (follicular adenoma/carcinoma). One and three month studies in the rat have suggested that these results are linked to a nicardipine-induced reduction in plasma thyroxine (T4) levels with a consequent increase in plasma levels of thyroid stimulating hormone (TSH). Chronic elevation of TSH is known to cause hyperstimulation of the thyroid. In rats on an iodine deficient diet, nicardipine administration for one month was associated with thyroid hyperplasia that was prevented by T4 supplementation. Mice treated with nicardipine in the diet (at concentrations calculated to provide daily dosage levels of up to 100 mg/kg/day) for up to 18 months showed no evidence of neoplasia of any tissue and no evidence of thyroid changes. There was no evidence of thyroid pathology in dogs treated with up to 25 mg nicardipine/kg/day for one year and no evidence of effects of nicardipine on thyroid function (plasma T4 and TSH) in man.

There was no evidence of a mutagenic potential of nicardipine in a battery of genotoxicity tests conducted on microbial indicator organisms, in micronucleus tests in mice and hamsters, or in a sister chromatid exchange study in hamsters.

No impairment of fertility was seen in male or female rats administered nicardipine at oral doses as high as 100 mg/kg/day (50 times the 40 mg TID maximum recommended antianginal or antihypertensive dose in man, assuming a patient weight of 60 kg).

Pregnancy Pregnancy Category C

Nicardipine was embryocidal when administered orally to pregnant Japanese White rabbits, during organogenesis, at 150 mg/kg/day (a dose associated with marked body weight gain suppression in the treated doe) but not at 50 mg/kg/day (25 times the maximum recommended antianginal or antihypertensive dose in man). No adverse effects on the fetus were observed when New Zealand albino rabbits were treated, during organogenesis, with up to 100 mg nicardipine/kg/day (a dose associated with significant mortality in the treated doe). In pregnant rats administered nicardipine orally at up to 100 mg/kg/day (50 times the maximum recommended human dose) there was no evidence of embryolethality or teratogenicity. However, dystocia, reduced birth weights, reduced neonatal survival and reduced neonatal weight gain were noted. There are no adequate and well-controlled studies in pregnant women. CARDENE® should be used during pregnancy only if the potential benefit justifies the potential risk to the fetus.

Nursing Mothers

Studies in rats have shown significant concentrations of CARDENE in maternal milk following oral administration. For this reason it is recommended that women who wish to breast-feed should not take this drug.

Pediatric Use

Safety and efficacy in patients under the age of 18 have not been established.

Use in the Elderly

Pharmacokinetic parameters did not differ between elderly hypertensive patients (≥65 years) and healthy controls after one week of CARDENE treatment at 20 mg TID. Plasma CARDENE concentrations in elderly hypertensive patients were similar to plasma concentrations in healthy young adult subjects when CARDENE was administered at doses of 10, 20 and 30 mg TID, suggesting that the pharmacokinetics of CARDENE are similar in young and elderly hypertensive patients. No significant differences in responses to CARDENE have been observed in elderly patients and the general adult population of patients who participated in clinical studies.

ADVERSE REACTIONS

In multiple-dose U.S. and foreign controlled short-term (up to three months) studies 1,910 patients received CARDENE alone or in combination with other drugs. In these studies adverse events were reported spontaneously; adverse experiences were generally not serious but occasionally required dosage adjustment and about 10% of patients left the studies prematurely because of them. Peak responses were not observed to be associated with adverse effects during clinical trials, but physicians should be aware that adverse effects associated with decreases in blood pressure (tachycardia, hypotension, etc.) could occur around the time of the peak effect. Most adverse effects were expected consequences of the vasodilator effects of CARDENE.

Angina

The incidence rates of adverse effects in anginal patients were derived from multicenter, controlled clinical trials. Following are the rates of adverse effects for CARDENE (N = 520) and placebo (N = 310), respectively, that occurred in 0.4% of patients or more. These represent events considered probably drug-related by the investigator (except for certain cardiovascular events which were recorded in a different category). Where the frequency of adverse effects for CARDENE and placebo is similar, causal relationship is uncertain. The only dose-related effects were pedal edema and increased angina.

Percent of Patients with Adverse Effects in Controlled Studies
(Incidence of discontinuations shown in parentheses)

Adverse Experience	CARDENE (N = 520)		PLACEBO (N = 310)	
Pedal Edema	7.1	(0)	0.3	(0)
Dizziness	6.9	(1.2)	0.6	(0)
Headache	6.4	(0.6)	2.6	(0)
Asthenia	5.8	(0.4)	2.6	(0)
Flushing	5.6	(0.4)	1.0	(0)
Increased Angina	5.6	(3.5)	4.2	(1.9)
Palpitations	3.3	(0.4)	0.3	(0)
Nausea	1.9	(0)	0.3	(0)
Dyspepsia	1.5	(0.6)	0.6	(0.3)
Dry Mouth	1.4	(0)	0.3	(0)
Somnolence	1.4	(0)	1.0	(0)
Rash	1.2	(0.2)	0.3	(0)
Tachycardia	1.2	(0.2)	0.6	(0)
Myalgia	1.0	(0)	0.0	(0)
Other edema	1.0	(0.2)	0.3	(0)
Paresthesia	0.8	(0.6)	0.6	(0)
Sustained Tachycardia	0.8	(0.2)	0.6	(0)
Syncope	0.6	(0)	0.0	(0)
Constipation	0.6	(0.6)	0.6	(0)
Dyspnea	0.6	(0)	0.0	(0)
Abnormal ECG	0.6	(0)	0.0	(0)
Malaise	0.6	(0)	0.0	(0)
Nervousness	0.6	(0)	0.3	(0)
Tremor	0.6	(0)	0.0	(0)

In addition, adverse events were observed which are not readily distinguishable from the natural history of the atherosclerotic vascular disease in these patients. Adverse events in this category each occurred in <0.4% of patients receiving CARDENE and included myocardial infarction, atrial fibrillation, exertional hypotension, pericarditis, heart block, cerebral ischemia and ventricular tachycardia. It is possible that some of these events were drug-related.

Hypertension

The incidence rates of adverse effects in hypertensive patients were derived from multicenter, controlled clinical trials. Following are the rates of adverse effects for CARDENE (N = 1390) and placebo (N = 211), respectively, that occurred in 0.4% of patients or more. These represent events considered probably drug-related by the investigator. Where the frequency of adverse effects for CARDENE and placebo is similar, causal relationship is uncertain. The only dose-related effect was pedal edema.

Percent of Patients with Adverse Effects in Controlled Studies
(Incidence of discontinuations shown in parentheses)

Adverse Experience	CARDENE (N = 1390)	PLACEBO (N = 211)
Flushing	9.7 (2.1)	2.8 (0)
Headache	8.2 (2.6)	4.7 (0)
Pedal Edema	8.0 (1.8)	0.9 (0)
Asthenia	4.2 (1.7)	0.5 (0)
Palpitations	4.1 (1.0)	0.0 (0)
Dizziness	4.0 (1.8)	0.0 (0)
Tachycardia	3.4 (1.2)	0.5 (0)
Nausea	2.2 (0.9)	0.9 (0)
Somnolence	1.1 (0.1)	0.0 (0)
Dyspepsia	0.8 (0.3)	0.0 (0)
Insomnia	0.6 (0.1)	0.5 (0)
Malaise	0.6 (0.1)	0.0 (0)
Other edema	0.6 (0.3)	1.4 (0)
Abnormal dreams	0.4 (0)	0.0 (0)
Dry mouth	0.4 (0.1)	0.0 (0)
Nocturia	0.4 (0)	0.0 (0)
Rash	0.4 (0.4)	0.0 (0)
Vomiting	0.4 (0.4)	0.0 (0)

Rare Events

The following rare adverse events have been reported in clinical trials or the literature:

Body as a Whole: infection, allergic reaction
Cardiovascular: hypotension, postural hypotension, atypical chest pain, peripheral vascular disorder, ventricular extrasystoles, ventricular tachycardia
Digestive: sore throat, abnormal liver chemistries
Musculoskeletal: arthralgia
Nervous: hot flashes, vertigo, hyperkinesia, impotence, depression, confusion, anxiety
Respiratory: rhinitis, sinusitis
Special Senses: tinnitus, abnormal vision, blurred vision
Urogenital: increased urinary frequency

OVERDOSAGE

Overdosage with a 600 mg single dose (15 to 30 times normal clinical dose) has been reported. Marked hypotension (blood pressure unobtainable) and bradycardia (heart rate 20 bpm in normal sinus rhythm) occurred, along with drowsiness, confusion and slurred speech. Supportive treatment with a vasopressor resulted in gradual improvement with normal vital signs approximately 9 hours post treatment.

Based on results obtained in laboratory animals, overdosage may cause systemic hypotension, bradycardia (following initial tachycardia) and progressive atrio-ventricular conduction block. Reversible hepatic function abnormalities and sporadic focal hepatic necrosis were noted in some animal species receiving very large doses of nicardipine.

For treatment of overdosage standard measures (for example, evacuation of gastric contents, elevation of extremities, attention to circulating fluid volume and urine output) including monitoring of cardiac and respiratory functions should be implemented. The patient should be positioned so as to avoid cerebral anoxia. Frequent blood pressure determinations are essential. Vasopressors are clinically indicated for patients exhibiting profound hypotension. Intravenous calcium gluconate may help reverse the effects of calcium entry blockade.

DOSAGE AND ADMINISTRATION

Angina

The dose should be individually titrated for each patient beginning with 20 mg three times daily. Doses in the range of 20-40 mg three times a day have been shown to be effective. At least three days should be allowed before increasing the CARDENE dose to ensure achievement of steady state plasma drug concentrations.

Concomitant Use With Other Antianginal Agents
1. Sublingual NTG may be taken as required to abort acute anginal attacks during CARDENE therapy.
2. Prophylactic Nitrate Therapy - CARDENE may be safely coadministered with short- and long-acting nitrates.
3. Beta-blockers - CARDENE may be safely coadministered with beta-blockers. (See DRUG INTERACTIONS.)

Hypertension

The dose of CARDENE should be individually adjusted according to the blood pressure response beginning with 20 mg three times daily. The effective doses in clinical trials have ranged from 20 mg to 40 mg three times daily. **To assess the adequacy of blood pressure response, the blood pressure should be measured at trough (8 hours after dosing). Because of the prominent peak effects of nicardipine, blood pressure should also be measured 1-2 hours after dosing, particularly during initiation of therapy.** (See PRECAUTIONS: Blood Pressure.) At least three days should be allowed before increasing the CARDENE dose to ensure achievement of steady state plasma drug concentrations.

Concomitant use with other Antihypertensive Agents
1. Diuretics - CARDENE may be safely coadministered with thiazide diuretics.
2. Beta-blockers - CARDENE may be safely coadministered with beta-blockers. (See DRUG INTERACTIONS.)

Special Patient Populations

Renal Insufficiency - although there is no evidence that CARDENE impairs renal function, careful dose titration beginning with 20 mg TID is advised. (See PRECAUTIONS.)

Hepatic Insufficiency - CARDENE should be administered cautiously in patients with severely impaired hepatic function. A suggested starting dose of 20 mg twice a day is advised with individual titration based on clinical findings maintaining the twice a day schedule. (See PRECAUTIONS.)

Congestive Heart Failure - Caution is advised when titrating CARDENE dosage in patients with congestive heart failure. (See WARNINGS.)

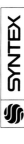
CYTOVENE®
(ganciclovir sodium)
Sterile Powder

FOR INTRAVENOUS INFUSION ONLY

THE CLINICAL TOXICITY OF **CYTOVENE** INCLUDES GRANULOCYTOPENIA AND THROMBOCYTOPENIA. IN ANIMAL STUDIES **CYTOVENE** WAS CARCINOGENIC, TERATOGENIC, AND CAUSED ASPERMATOGENESIS. **CYTOVENE** IS INDICATED FOR USE *ONLY* IN IMMUNOCOMPROMISED PATIENTS WITH CYTOMEGALOVIRUS (CMV) RETINITIS.

DESCRIPTION

CYTOVENE is the brand name for ganciclovir sodium, an antiviral drug active against cytomegalovirus. Reconstituted CYTOVENE Sterile Powder is for intravenous administration only. Each vial of CYTOVENE Sterile Powder contains the equivalent of 500 mg ganciclovir as the sodium salt (46 mg sodium). All doses in this insert are specified in terms of ganciclovir. The chemical name of ganciclovir sodium is 9-(1,3-dihydroxy-2-propoxymethyl) guanine, monosodium salt, and it has the following structure:

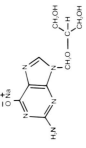

CYTOVENE is manufactured as a sterile lyophilized powder. Reconstitution with 10 mL of Sterile Water for Injection, USP, yields a solution with pH 11 and a ganciclovir concentration of approximately 50 mg/mL. Further dilution in an appropriate intravenous solution must be performed before infusion (see DOSAGE AND ADMINISTRATION).

CLINICAL PHARMACOLOGY

Virology

Ganciclovir is a synthetic nucleoside analogue of 2'-deoxyguanosine that inhibits replication of herpesviruses both *in vitro* and *in vivo*. Sensitive human viruses include cytomegalovirus (CMV), herpes simplex virus -1 and -2 (HSV-1, HSV-2), Epstein-Barr virus (EBV) and varicella zoster virus (VZV). Clinical studies have been limited to assessment of efficacy in patients with CMV infection.

Median effective inhibitory doses (ED$_{50}$) of ganciclovir for human CMV isolates tested *in vitro* in several cell lines ranged from 0.2 to 3.0 μg/mL. The relationship between *in vitro* sensitivity of CMV to ganciclovir and clinical response has not been established. CYTOVENE inhibits mammalian cell proliferation *in vitro* at higher concentrations (10 to 60 μg/mL) with bone marrow colony forming cells being the most sensitive (ID$_{50}$ ≥ 10 μg/mL) of those cell types tested.

Available evidence indicates that upon entry into host cells, cytomegaloviruses induce one or more cellular kinases that phosphorylate ganciclovir to its triphosphate. It has been shown that there is approximately a 10-fold greater concentration of ganciclovir-triphosphate in CMV-infected cells than in uninfected cells, indicating a preferential phosphorylation of ganciclovir in virus-infected cells. *In vitro*, ganciclovir-triphosphate is catabolized slowly, with 60 to 70% of the original level remaining in the infected cells 18 hours after removal of ganciclovir from the extracellular medium.[1] The antiviral activity of ganciclovir-triphosphate is believed to be the result of inhibition of viral DNA synthesis by two known modes: (1) competitive inhibition of viral DNA polymerases (2) direct incorporation into viral DNA, resulting in eventual termination of viral DNA elongation. The cellular DNA polymerase alpha is also inhibited, but at a higher concentration than required for viral DNA polymerase.

Ganciclovir has shown antiviral activity *in vivo* in several animal CMV infection models. Both normal and immunosuppressed mice had reduced titers of murine CMV when treated with ganciclovir at 5 to 50 mg/kg/day.[2] Normal mice had increased survival as well, when treated with doses of 3 mg/kg/day. Immunosuppressed mice did not show increased survival until they received doses of at least 10 mg/kg/day.[3] In guinea pigs infected with cavian CMV and treated with ganciclovir at 50 mg/kg/day for 7 days, viral titers in the salivary glands were reduced approximately 50% at day 28 post-infection as compared to sham-treated controls.[4]

Of 314 immunocompromised patients enrolled in an open label study of the treatment of life- or sight-threatening CMV disease, 121 patients were identified who had a positive culture for CMV within 7 days prior to treatment and had sequential viral cultures after treatment with CYTOVENE.[5] Post-treatment virologic response was defined as conversion to culture negativity, or a greater than 100-fold decrease in CMV infectious units, as shown in the following table:

Virologic Response

Culture Source	No. Patients Cultured	No. (%) Patients Responding	Median Days to Response
Urine	107	93 (87)	8
Blood	41	34 (83)	8
Throat	21	19 (90)	7
Semen	6	6 (100)	15

Emergence of viral resistance has been reported based on *in vitro* sensitivity testing of CMV isolates from patients receiving CYTOVENE treatment.[6] The prevalence of resistant isolates is unknown, and there is a possibility that some patients may be infected with strains of CMV resistant to ganciclovir. Therefore, the possibility of viral resistance should be considered in patients who show poor clinical response or experience persistent viral excretion during therapy.

Pharmacokinetics

The pharmacokinetics of CYTOVENE have been evaluated in immunocompromised patients with serious CMV disease. Twenty-two patients with normal renal function, enrolled in open-label treatment at different study centers, received 5 mg/kg doses of CYTOVENE, each dose infused intravenously over one hour. The plasma level of ganciclovir at the end of the first one hour infusion (Cmax) was 8.3 ± 4.0 μg/mL (mean ± SD) and the plasma level 11 hours after the start of infusion (Cmin) was 0.56 ± 0.66 μg/mL. The plasma half-life was 2.9 ± 1.3 hours and the systemic clearance was 3.64 ± 1.86 mL/kg/min (approximately 250 mL/min/1.73M²). Dose-independent kinetics were demonstrated over the range of 1.6 to 5.0 mg/kg. Multiple-dose kinetics were measured in eight patients with normal renal function who received CYTOVENE* (ganciclovir sodium) Sterile Powder, 5 mg/kg twice daily for 12-14 days. After the first dose and after multiple dosing, plasma levels of ganciclovir at the end of infusion were 7.1 μg/mL (3.1 to 14.0 μg/mL) and 9.5 μg/mL (2.7 to 24.2 μg/mL), respectively. At 7 hours after infusion, plasma levels after the first dose were 0.85 μg/mL (0.2 to 1.8 μg/mL) and were 1.2 μg/mL (0.6 to 1.8 μg/mL) after multiple dosing.

Renal excretion of unchanged drug by glomerular filtration is the major route of elimination of CYTOVENE. In patients with normal renal function, more than 90% of the administered CYTOVENE was recovered unmetabolized in the urine. The pharmacokinetic analysis in 10 patients with renal impairment showed that in 4 patients with mild impairment (creatinine clearance 50 to 79 mL/min/1.73M²) the systemic clearance of CYTOVENE was 128 ± 63 mL/min/1.73M², and the plasma half-life was 4.6 ± 1.4 hours. In 3 patients with moderate impairment (creatinine clearance 25 to 49 mL/min/1.73M²) the systemic clearance of CYTOVENE was 57 ± 8 mL/min/1.73M², and the plasma half-life was 4.4 ± 0.4 hours. In 3 patients with severe impairment (creatinine clearance less than 25 mL/min/1.73M²) the systemic clearance was 30 ± 13 mL/min/1.73M², and the plasma half-life was 10.7 ± 5.7 hours. There was positive correlation between systemic clearance of CYTOVENE and creatinine clearance (r = 0.90).

Data from 4 patients with severe renal impairment showed that hemodialysis reduced plasma drug levels by approximately 50%.

BECAUSE THE MAJOR EXCRETION PATHWAY FOR CYTOVENE* IS RENAL, DOSAGE MUST BE REDUCED ACCORDING TO CREATININE CLEARANCE. FOR DOSING INSTRUCTIONS IN RENAL IMPAIRMENT, REFER TO THE SECTION ON DOSAGE AND ADMINISTRATION.

There is limited evidence to suggest that ganciclovir crosses the blood-brain barrier. Cerebrospinal fluid (CSF) concentrations have been measured in three patients who received 2.5 mg/kg ganciclovir intravenously q8 or q12 hours. The results are shown in the following table:

CSF Concentrations[7,8]

Patient	CSF Conc. (μg/mL)	Plasma Conc. (μg/mL)	Hr after dose	CSF/Plasma Ratio
1	0.62	0.92*	5.67	67
	0.68	2.20*	3.5	31
	0.51	1.96*	2.75	26
2	0.50	2.05*	0.25	24
3	0.31	0.44	5.5	70

*Estimation (model-predicted values)

Binding of CYTOVENE to plasma proteins is 1-2%. Drug interactions involving binding site displacement are not expected.

INDICATIONS AND USAGE

CYTOVENE is indicated for the treatment of CMV retinitis in immunocompromised individuals, including patients with acquired immunodeficiency syndrome (AIDS). SAFETY AND EFFICACY OF **CYTOVENE** HAVE NOT BEEN ESTABLISHED FOR CONGENITAL OR NEONATAL CMV DISEASE; NOR FOR TREATMENT OF OTHER CMV INFECTIONS (E.G., PNEUMONITIS, COLITIS); NOR FOR USE IN NON-IMMUNOCOMPROMISED INDIVIDUALS.

The diagnosis of CMV retinitis is ophthalmologic and should be made by indirect ophthalmoscopy. Other conditions in the differential diagnosis of CMV retinitis include candidiasis, toxoplasmosis, histoplasmosis, retinal scars, and cotton wool spots, any of which may produce a retinal appearance similar to CMV. For this reason it is essential that the diagnosis of CMV be established by an ophthalmologist familiar with the retinal presentation of these conditions. The diagnosis of CMV retinitis may be supported by culture of CMV from urine, blood, throat, or other sites, but a negative CMV culture does not rule out CMV retinitis.

In most studies conducted with CYTOVENE, treatment was begun with a BID dosage regimen (5 mg/kg/dose) for the first 2 to 3 weeks, followed by a once-daily regimen (maintenance treatment) to maintain viral suppression. Patients who experienced progression of retinitis while receiving maintenance treatment were retreated with the BID regimen (see DOSAGE AND ADMINISTRATION).

In a retrospective, non-randomized, single-center analysis[9,10] of 41 patients with AIDS and CMV retinitis, treatment with CYTOVENE resulted in a significant delay in median time to first retinitis progression compared to untreated controls (71 days from diagnosis versus 29 days from diagnosis). Patients in this series received induction treatment of CYTOVENE 5 mg/kg BID for 14-21 days followed by maintenance treatment with either 5 mg/kg once per day, seven days per week or 6 mg/kg once per day, five days each week.

CONTRAINDICATIONS

CYTOVENE is contraindicated in patients with hypersensitivity to ganciclovir or acyclovir.

WARNINGS

Approximately 40% of 522 immunocompromised patients with serious CMV infections who received intravenous CYTOVENE developed granulocytopenia (neutropenia, i.e., neutrophil count less than 1,000 cells/mm³). CYTOVENE should, therefore, be used with caution in patients with pre-existing cytopenias, or with a history of cytopenic reactions to other drugs, chemicals or irradiation. Granulocytopenia usually occurs during the first or second week of treatment, but may occur at any time during treatment. Cell counts usually begin to recover within 3 to 7 days of discontinuing drug. *CYTOVENE should not be administered if the absolute neutrophil count is less than 500 cells/mm³ or the platelet count is less than 25,000/mm³.*

Thrombocytopenia (platelet count <50,000/mm³) was observed in approximately 20% of the same 522 patients treated with CYTOVENE. Patients with iatrogenic immunosuppression were more likely to develop thrombocytopenia than patients with AIDS (46% versus 14% of cases).

Animal data indicate that administration of CYTOVENE causes inhibition of spermatogenesis and subsequent infertility. These effects were reversible at lower doses and irreversible at higher doses (see Carcinogenesis, Mutagenesis, Impairment of Fertility section in PRECAUTIONS). Although data in humans have not been obtained regarding this effect, *it is considered probable that intravenous CYTOVENE at the recommended doses causes temporary or permanent inhibition of spermatogenesis. Animal data also indicate that suppression of fertility in females may occur.*

Because of the mutagenic potential of CYTOVENE, women of childbearing potential should be advised to use effective contraception during treatment. Similarly, male patients should be advised to practice barrier contraception during and for at least 90 days following treatment with CYTOVENE.

PRECAUTIONS

General

In clinical studies with CYTOVENE, the maximum single dose administered was 6 mg/kg by intravenous infusion over one hour. It is likely that larger doses, or more rapid infusions, would result in increased toxicity.

Administration of CYTOVENE by intravenous infusion should be accompanied by adequate hydration, since CYTOVENE is excreted by the kidneys and normal clearance depends on adequate renal function. **IF RENAL FUNCTION IS IMPAIRED, DOSAGE ADJUSTMENTS ARE REQUIRED.** Such adjustments should be based on measured or estimated creatinine clearance (see DOSAGE AND ADMINISTRATION).

Initially reconstituted CYTOVENE solutions have a high pH (pH 11). Despite further dilution in intravenous fluids, phlebitis and/or pain may occur at the site of intravenous infusion. Care must be taken to infuse solutions containing CYTOVENE only into veins with adequate blood flow to permit rapid dilution and distribution (see DOSAGE AND ADMINISTRATION).

Information for Patients

CYTOVENE® (ganciclovir sodium) Sterile Powder is not a cure for CMV retinitis, and immunocompromised patients may continue to experience progression of retinitis during or following treatment. Patients should be advised to have ophthalmologic follow-up examinations at a minimum of every six weeks while being treated with CYTOVENE. (Many patients will require more frequent follow-up.) They should be informed that the major toxicities of ganciclovir are granulocytopenia and thrombocytopenia and that dose modifications may be required, including possible discontinuation. The importance of close monitoring of blood counts while on therapy should be emphasized.

Patients with AIDS may be receiving zidovudine (Retrovir). They should be counseled that treatment with zidovudine or CYTOVENE, and especially the combination, can result in severe granulocytopenia. Therefore, it is recommended that the two drugs not be given concomitantly.

Patients should be advised that CYTOVENE has caused decreased sperm production in animals and may cause infertility in humans. Women of childbearing potential should be advised that CYTOVENE causes birth defects in animals and should not be used during pregnancy. Women of childbearing potential should be advised to use effective contraception during CYTOVENE treatment. Similarly, men should be advised to practice barrier contraception during and for at least 90 days following CYTOVENE treatment.

Patients should be advised that CYTOVENE causes tumors in animals. Although there is no information from human studies, CYTOVENE should be considered a potential carcinogen.

Laboratory Testing

Due to the frequency of granulocytopenia and thrombocytopenia in patients receiving CYTOVENE (see ADVERSE REACTIONS), it is recommended that neutrophil counts and platelet counts be performed every two days during BID dosing of CYTOVENE and at least weekly thereafter. Neutrophil counts should be monitored daily in patients in whom CYTOVENE or other nucleoside analogues have previously resulted in leukopenia, or in whom neutrophil counts are less than 1,000 cells/mm³ at the beginning of treatment. Because dosing must be modified in patients with renal impairment, patients should have serum creatinine or creatinine clearance monitored at least once every two weeks.

Drug Interactions

It is possible that probenecid, as well as other drugs that inhibit renal tubular secretion or resorption, may reduce renal clearance of CYTOVENE. It is also possible that drugs that inhibit replication of rapidly dividing cell populations such as bone marrow, spermatogonia, and germinal layers of skin and gastrointestinal mucosa may have additive toxicity when administered concomitantly with CYTOVENE. Therefore, drugs such as dapsone, pentamidine, flucytosine, vincristine, vinblastine, adriamycin, amphotericin B, trimethoprim/sulfa combinations or other nucleoside analogues, should be considered for concomitant use with CYTOVENE only if the potential benefits are judged to outweigh the risks.

Patients with AIDS may be receiving, or have received, treatment with zidovudine (Retrovir). *Because both zidovudine and CYTOVENE can cause granulocytopenia, it is recommended that these two drugs not be given concomitantly.* Data from a small number of patients indicate that treatment with ganciclovir plus zidovudine at the recommended doses is not tolerated.

Generalized seizures have been reported in six patients who received CYTOVENE and imipenem-cilastatin. These drugs should not be used concomitantly with CYTOVENE unless the potential benefits outweigh the risks.

Carcinogenesis, Mutagenesis, Impairment of Fertility

Ganciclovir was carcinogenic in the mouse after daily oral doses of 20 and 1000 mg/kg/day. The principally affected tissues at the dose of 1000 mg/kg/day were the preputial gland in males, forestomach (nonglandular mucosa) in males and females, and reproductive tissues and liver in females. At doses of 20 mg/kg/day, slightly increased tumor incidences occurred in the preputial and harderian glands in males, forestomach in males and females, and liver in females. All ganciclovir-induced tumors were of epithelial or vascular origin, except for histiocytic sarcoma of the liver. No carcinogenic effect occurred at the dose of 1 mg/kg/day. The preputial and clitoral glands, forestomach, and harderian glands of mice do not have human counterparts. However, CYTOVENE should be considered a potential carcinogen in humans.

Ganciclovir was mutagenic in mouse lymphoma cells and caused chromosomal damage *in vitro* in human lymphocytes and *in vivo* in mice.

Ganciclovir caused decreased mating behavior, decreased fertility, and increased embryolethality in female mice at doses approximately equivalent to the recommended human dose (calculated on the basis of body surface area). Ganciclovir caused decreased fertility in male mice and hypospermatogenesis in rats and dogs at doses equivalent to or less than the recommended human dose.

Pregnancy: Category C

CYTOVENE has been shown to be teratogenic in rabbits and embryotoxic in mice when given in doses approximately equivalent to the recommended human dose (calculated on the basis of body surface area). The adverse effects observed in mice were maternal/fetal toxicity and embryolethality. In rabbits, the effects were: fetal growth retardation, embryolethality, teratogenicity, and/or maternal toxicity. Teratogenic changes included cleft palate, anophthalmia/microphthalmia, aplastic organs (kidney and pancreas), hydrocephaly, and brachygnathia.

It is therefore expected that CYTOVENE may be teratogenic and/or embryotoxic at the dose levels recommended for human use. There are no adequate and well-controlled studies in pregnant women. CYTOVENE should be used during pregnancy only if the potential benefit justifies the potential risk to the fetus.

Nursing Mothers

It is not known if CYTOVENE is excreted in human milk. Because many drugs are excreted in human milk and because of the potential for serious adverse reactions from ganciclovir in nursing infants, mothers should be instructed to discontinue nursing if they are receiving CYTOVENE. The minimum interval before nursing can safely be resumed after the last dose of CYTOVENE is unknown.

Daily intravenous doses of 90 mg/kg administered to female mice prior to mating, during gestation, and during lactation caused hypoplasia of the testes and seminal vesicles in the month-old male offspring, as well as pathologic changes in the non-glandular region of the stomach.

Pediatric Use

THE USE OF CYTOVENE IN CHILDREN WARRANTS EXTREME CAUTION DUE TO THE PROBABILITY OF LONG-TERM CARCINOGENICITY AND REPRODUCTIVE TOXICITY. ADMINISTRATION TO CHILDREN SHOULD BE UNDERTAKEN ONLY AFTER CAREFUL EVALUATION AND ONLY IF THE POTENTIAL BENEFITS OF TREATMENT OUTWEIGH THE RISKS.

There has been very limited clinical experience in treating cytomegalovirus retinitis in patients under the age of 12 years. Two children (ages 9 and 5 years) showed improvement or stabilization of retinitis for 23 and 9 months, respectively. These children received induction treatment with 2.5 mg/kg TID followed by maintenance therapy with 6-6.5 mg/kg once per day, five to seven days per week. When retinitis progressed during once daily maintenance therapy, both children were treated with the 5 mg/kg BID regimen. Two other children (ages 2.5 and 4 years) who received similar induction regimens showed only partial or no response to treatment. Another child, a six year old with T-cell dysfunction, showed stabilization of retinitis for 3 months while receiving continuous infusions of CYTOVENE at doses of 2-5 mg/kg/24 hours. Continuous infusion treatment was discontinued due to granulocytopenia. Pharmacokinetic data have not been obtained in pediatric patients.

Adverse events reported in 120 immunocompromised children with serious CMV infections receiving ganciclovir were similar to those reported in adults. Granulocytopenia (17%) and thrombocytopenia (10%) were the most common adverse events reported.

Use in Patients with Renal Impairment

CYTOVENE should be used with caution in patients with impaired renal function because the plasma half-life and peak plasma levels of CYTOVENE will be increased due to reduced renal clearance (see DOSAGE AND ADMINISTRATION).

Data from 4 patients indicate that CYTOVENE plasma levels are reduced approximately 50% following hemodialysis.

Use in the Elderly

No studies of the efficacy or safety of CYTOVENE in elderly patients have been conducted. Since elderly individuals frequently have reduced glomerular filtration, particular attention should be paid to assessing renal function before and during CYTOVENE administration (see DOSAGE AND ADMINISTRATION).

ADVERSE REACTIONS

During clinical trials, CYTOVENE® (ganciclovir sodium) Sterile Powder was withdrawn or interrupted in approximately 32% of patients because of adverse events. In some instances treatment was restarted and the reappearance of adverse events again necessitated withdrawal or interruption.

The most frequent adverse events seen in patients treated with CYTOVENE involved the hematopoietic system. Granulocytopenia (defined as an absolute neutrophil count less than 1,000 cells/mm^3) occurred in approximately 40% and thrombocytopenia (defined as a platelet count below 50,000/mm^3) occurred in approximately 20% of the patients. In most cases, withdrawal of CYTOVENE resulted in increased neutrophil or platelet counts.

While granulocytopenia was generally reversible with discontinuation of treatment, some patients experienced irreversible neutropenia or died with severe bacterial or fungal infections during neutropenic episodes.

Adverse events other than granulocytopenia and thrombocytopenia were reported as "probably related", "probably not related", and "unknown" in relationship to CYTOVENE therapy. Evaluation of these reports was difficult because of the protean manifestations of the underlying disease, and because most patients received numerous concomitant medications.

Retinal detachments have been observed in patients with CMV retinitis both before and after initiation of CYTOVENE therapy. The relationship of retinal detachments to CYTOVENE therapy is unknown. Patients with CMV retinitis should have frequent ophthalmologic evaluations to monitor the status of their retinitis and detect any other retinal lesions.

Other than leukopenia and thrombocytopenia, the most frequent adverse events observed in over 5,000 patients who received CYTOVENE were anemia, fever, rash, and abnormal liver function values, each of which was reported in approximately 2% of treated patients. Adverse events that were thought to be possibly related to drug and occurred in 1% or fewer patients who received CYTOVENE were:

Body as a Whole: chills, edema, infections, malaise

Cardiovascular System: arrhythmia, hypertension, hypotension

Central Nervous System: abnormal thoughts or dreams, ataxia, coma, confusion, dizziness, headache, nervousness, paresthesia, psychosis, somnolence, tremor. (Overall, neurologic system events occurred in 5% of patients.)

Digestive System: nausea, vomiting, anorexia, diarrhea, hemorrhage, abdominal pain

Hematologic System: eosinophilia

Laboratory Abnormalities: decrease in blood glucose

Respiratory System: dyspnea

Skin and Appendages: alopecia, pruritus, urticaria

Urogenital System: hematuria, increased serum creatinine, increased blood urea nitrogen (BUN)

Injection Site: inflammation, pain, phlebitis

OVERDOSAGE

Overdosage with CYTOVENE has been reported in five patients. In three of these patients, no adverse events were observed after the overdosage. (The doses received were: 7 doses of 22 mg/kg over a 3-day period, 9 mg/kg BID for 3 days, and 2 doses of 500 mg given to a 21 month old child.)

Neutropenia was reported following overdoses in two patients: one who had a history of bone marrow suppression prior to treatment and who received CYTOVENE 5 mg/kg BID for 14 days followed by treatment with 8 mg/kg given as single daily doses for 4 days, and one patient who received a single dose of 1,675 mg (approximately 24 mg/kg). In both cases the neutropenia was reversible (17 days and 1 day, respectively), following discontinuation of CYTOVENE.

Single intravenous doses of ganciclovir given to mice and dogs caused mortality at high dosages. The median lethal acute intravenous dose of ganciclovir was 900 mg/kg in mice and between 150 and 500 mg/kg in dogs. Toxic manifestations observed in mice and dogs given very high single doses of CYTOVENE (500 mg/kg) included emesis, hypersalivation, anorexia, bloody diarrhea, inactivity, cytopenia, elevated blood urea nitrogen, elevated liver function test results, testicular atrophy and death.

Hemodialysis and hydration may be of benefit in reducing drug plasma levels in patients who receive an overdosage of CYTOVENE.

DOSAGE AND ADMINISTRATION

CAUTION – DO NOT ADMINISTER CYTOVENE BY RAPID OR BOLUS INTRAVENOUS INJECTION. THE TOXICITY OF *CYTOVENE* MAY BE INCREASED AS A RESULT OF EXCESSIVE PLASMA LEVELS.

CAUTION – INTRAMUSCULAR OR SUBCUTANEOUS INJECTION OF RECONSTITUTED *CYTOVENE* MAY RESULT IN SEVERE TISSUE IRRITATION DUE TO HIGH PH (11).

Dosage
THE RECOMMENDED DOSAGE, FREQUENCY, OR INFUSION RATES SHOULD NOT BE EXCEEDED.

Induction Treatment. The recommended initial dose of CYTOVENE for patients with normal renal function is 5 mg/kg (given intravenously at a constant rate over 1 hour) every 12 hours for 14-21 days.

Maintenance Treatment. Following induction treatment the recommended dose of CYTOVENE is 5 mg/kg given as an intravenous infusion over one hour once per day on seven days each week, or 6 mg/kg once per day on five days each week. Patients who experience progression of retinitis while receiving maintenance therapy may be retreated with the BID regimen.

Patients should have frequent hematologic monitoring throughout treatment. CYTOVENE should not be administered if the neutrophil count falls below 500 cells/mm^3 or the platelet count falls below 25,000/mm^3.

RENAL IMPAIRMENT
For patients with impairment of renal function, refer to the table below for recommended doses during the induction phase of treatment, and adjust the dosing interval as indicated.

Creatinine Clearance* (mL/min)	CYTOVENE Dose (mg/kg)	Dosing Interval (hours)
>80	5.0	12
50-79	2.5	12
25-49	2.5	24
<25	1.25	24

*Creatinine clearance can be related to serum creatinine by the following formulae:

Creatinine clearance for males = $\dfrac{(140 - \text{age[yrs]}) \,(\text{body wt [kg]})}{(72) \,(\text{serum creatinine [mg/dL]})}$

Creatinine clearance for females = 0.85 × male value

The optimal maintenance dose for patients with renal impairment is not known. Physicians may elect to reduce the dose to 50% of the induction dose and monitor the patient for disease progression.

Only limited data are available on CYTOVENE® (ganciclovir sodium) Sterile Powder elimination in patients undergoing hemodialysis. Dosing for these patients should not exceed 1.25 mg/kg/24 hours. On days when hemodialysis is performed, the dose should be given shortly after the completion of the hemodialysis session, since hemodialysis has been shown to reduce plasma levels by approximately 50%. Neutrophil and platelet counts should be monitored daily.

PATIENT MONITORING

Due to the frequency of granulocytopenia and thrombocytopenia in patients receiving CYTOVENE (see ADVERSE REACTIONS), it is recommended that neutrophil counts and platelet counts be performed every two days during BID dosing of CYTOVENE and at least weekly thereafter. In patients in whom CYTOVENE or other nucleoside analogues have previously resulted in leukopenia, or in whom neutrophil counts are less than 1,000 cells/mm^3 at the beginning of treatment, neutrophil counts should be monitored daily. Because dosing must be modified in patients with renal impairment, all patients should have serum creatinine or creatinine clearance monitored at least once every two weeks.

REDUCTION OF DOSE

The most frequently reported adverse event following treatment with CYTOVENE is leukopenia/neutropenia, which occurs in approximately 40% of patients. Therefore, frequent white blood cell counts should be performed. Severe neutropenia (ANC less than 500/mm^3) or severe thrombocytopenia (platelets less than 25,000/mm^3) requires a dose interruption until evidence of marrow recovery is observed (ANC $\geq$ 750/mm^3).

Method of Preparation

Each 10 mL clear glass vial contains ganciclovir sodium equivalent to 500 mg of the free base form of CYTOVENE and 46 mg of sodium. The contents of the vial should be prepared for administration in the following manner:

1. Lyophilized CYTOVENE should be reconstituted by injecting 10 mL of Sterile Water for Injection, USP, into the vial.

DO NOT USE BACTERIOSTATIC WATER FOR INJECTION CONTAINING PARABENS. IT IS INCOMPATIBLE WITH CYTOVENE STERILE POWDER AND MAY CAUSE PRECIPITATION.

2. The vial should be shaken to dissolve the drug.

3. Reconstituted solution should be inspected visually for particulate matter and discoloration prior to proceeding with admixture preparation. If particulate matter or discoloration is observed, the vial should be discarded.

4. Reconstituted solution in the vial is stable at room temperature for 12 hours. It should not be refrigerated.

Admixture Preparation and Administration

Based on patient weight, the appropriate calculated dose volume should be removed from the vial (ganciclovir concentration 50 mg/mL) and added to an acceptable (see below) infusion fluid (typically 100 mL) for delivery over the course of one hour. Infusion concentrations greater than 10 mg/mL are not recommended. The following infusion fluids have been determined to be chemically and physically compatible with CYTOVENE: 0.9% Sodium Chloride, 5% Dextrose, Ringer's Injection, and Lactated Ringer's Injection, USP.

Note: Because non-bacteriostatic infusion fluid must be used with CYTOVENE, the infusion solution must be used within 24 hours of dilution to reduce the risk of bacterial contamination. The infusion solution should be refrigerated. Freezing is not recommended.

HANDLING AND DISPOSAL

Caution should be exercised in the handling and preparation of CYTOVENE solutions. CYTOVENE solutions are alkaline (pH 11). Avoid direct contact with the skin or mucous membranes. If such contact occurs, wash thoroughly with soap and water; rinse eyes thoroughly with plain water.

Because CYTOVENE shares some of the properties of anti-tumor agents (i.e. carcinogenicity and mutagenicity), consideration should be given to handling and disposal according to guidelines issued for antineoplastic drugs. Several guidelines on this subject have been published.[11-16]

There is no general agreement that all of the procedures recommended in the guidelines are necessary or appropriate.

HOW SUPPLIED

CYTOVENE® (ganciclovir sodium) Sterile Powder is supplied in 10 mL sterile vials, each containing ganciclovir sodium equivalent to 500 mg of ganciclovir, in cartons of 25 (NDC 0033-2903-48).

Store at room temperature. Avoid excessive heat, above 40°C (104°F).

CAUTION: Federal law prohibits dispensing without prescription.

REFERENCES

1. Smee D.F., Boehme R., Chernow M., et al: Intracellular metabolism and enzymatic phosphorylation of 9-(1,3-dihydroxy-2-propoxymethyl) guanine and acyclovir in herpes simplex virus-infected and uninfected cells. Biochemical Pharmacol 1985; 34:1049-1056.

2. Shanley J.D., Morningstar J., Jordan M.C.: Inhibition of murine cytomegalovirus lung infection and interstitial pneumonitis by acyclovir and 9-(1,3-dihydroxy-2-propoxymethyl) guanine. Antimicrob Agents Chemother 1985; 28: 172-175.

3. Wilson E.J, Medearis D.N. Jr, Hansen L.A., et al: 9-(1,3-dihydroxy-2-propoxymethyl) guanine prevents death but not immunity in murine cytomegalovirus-infected normal and immunosuppressed BALB/c mice. Antimicrob Agents Chemother 1987; 31:1017-1020.

4. Fong C.K.Y., Cohen S.D., McCormick S., Hsiung G.D.: Antiviral Effect of 9-(1,3-dihydroxy-2-propoxymethyl) guanine against cytomegalovirus infection in a guinea pig model. Antiviral Res 1987; 7: 11-23.

5. Buhles W.C., Mastre B.J., Tinker A.J., et al: Ganciclovir Treatment of Life-or Sight-Threatening Cytomegalovirus Infection: Experience in 314 Immunocompromised Patients. Rev Inf Dis 1988; 10:495-506.

6. Erice A., Chou S., Byron K.K., et al: Progressive disease due to ganciclovir-resistant cytomegalovirus in immunocompromised patients. N Eng J Med 1989; 320:289-293.

7. Fletcher C., Balfour H.: Evaluation of ganciclovir for cytomegalovirus disease. DICP, Ann Pharmacother 1989; 23:5-12.

8. Fletcher C., Sawchuk R., Chinnock B., et al: Human pharmacokinetics of the antiviral drug DHPG. Clin Pharmacol Ther 1986; 40: 281-286.

9. Jabs D., Enger E., Bartlett J.: Cytomegalovirus retinitis and acquired immunodeficiency syndrome. Arch Ophthalmol 1989; 107: 75-80.

10. Updated unpublished data on file with Syntex Corp.

11. Recommendations for the Safe Handling of Parenteral Antineoplastic Drugs. NIH Publication No. 83-2621. For sale by the Superintendent of Documents, U.S. Government Printing Office, Washington, D.C. 20402.

xxx

11. Recommendations for the Safe Handling of Parenteral Antineoplastic Drugs. NIH Publication No. 83-2621. For sale by the Superintendent of Documents, U.S. Government Printing Office, Washington, D.C. 20402.

12. AMA Council Report. Guidelines for Handling Parenteral Antineoplastics. *JAMA*, March 15, 1985.

13. National Study Commission on Cytotoxic Exposure-Recommendations for Handling Cytotoxic Agents. Available from Louis P. Jeffrey, Sc. D., Director of Pharmacy Services, Rhode Island Hospital, 593 Eddy Street, Providence, Rhode Island 02902.

14. Clinical Oncological Society of Australia: Guidelines and recommendations for safe handling of antineoplastic agents. *Med J Australia* 1:426-428 1983.

15. Jones R.B., et al. Safe handling of chemotherapeutic agents: A report from the Mount Sinai Medical Center, CA – *A Cancer Journal for Clinicians* Sept/Oct, 258-263 1983.

16. American Society of Hospital Pharmacists technical assistance bulletin on handling cytotoxic drugs in hospitals. *Am J Hosp Pharm* 42:131-137, 1985.

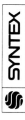

SYNTEX

Mfd. for Syntex Laboratories, Inc.
Palo Alto, CA 94304
Mfd. by Ben Venue Laboratories, Inc.
Bedford, Ohio 44146

02-2903-48-03
Revised August 1990

U.S. Patent No. 4,355,032; 4,507,305 and others.

FEMSTAT® PREFILL
(butoconazole nitrate)

Vaginal Cream 2%
Prefilled Applicator

DESCRIPTION

FEMSTAT Vaginal Cream contains butoconazole nitrate 2%, an imidazole derivative with antifungal activity. Its chemical name is ($\pm$)-1-[4-(*p*-Chlorophenyl)-2-[(2,6-dichlorophenyl) thio]butyl] imidazole mononitrate and it has the following chemical structure:

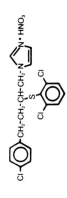

Butoconazole nitrate is a white to off-white crystalline powder with a molecular weight of 474.79. It is sparingly soluble in methanol; slightly soluble in chloroform, methylene chloride, acetone, and ethanol; very slightly soluble in ethyl acetate; and practically insoluble in water. It melts at about 159°C with decomposition.

FEMSTAT Vaginal Cream contains butoconazole nitrate 2% in a water-washable emollient cream of stearyl alcohol, propylene glycol, cetyl alcohol, sorbitan monostearate, glyceryl stearate (and) PEG-100 stearate, mineral oil, polysorbate 60, purified water, with methylparaben and propylparaben as preservatives.

CLINICAL PHARMACOLOGY

Butoconazole nitrate is an imidazole derivative that has fungicidal activity in vitro against *Candida*, *Trichophyton*, *Microsporum*, and *Epidermophyton*. It is also active against some gram positive bacteria. Clinically, it is highly effective against vaginal infections induced by strains of *Candida albicans*, *Candida tropicalis*, and other species of this genus.

The primary site of action of imidazoles appears to be the cell membrane. The permeability of the cell membrane is altered, resulting in a reduced osmotic resistance and viability of the fungus. The exact mechanism of antifungal activity of butoconazole nitrate is not known.

Following vaginal administration of butoconazole nitrate, 5.5% of the dose is absorbed on average. After vaginal administration peak plasma levels of the drug and its metabolites are attained at 24 hours and the plasma half-life is approximately 21-24 hours.

INDICATIONS AND USAGE

FEMSTAT Vaginal Cream is indicated for the local treatment of vulvovaginal mycotic infections caused by *Candida* species. The diagnosis should be confirmed by KOH smears and/or cultures.

FEMSTAT Vaginal Cream can be used in association with oral contraceptive and antibiotic therapy. FEMSTAT is effective in both non-pregnant and pregnant women but in pregnant women it should be used only during the second and third trimesters.

CONTRAINDICATIONS

FEMSTAT Vaginal Cream 2% is contraindicated in patients with a history of hypersensitivity to any of the components of the cream.

PRECAUTIONS

General:

If clinical symptoms persist, microbiological tests should be repeated to rule out other pathogens and to confirm the diagnosis.

If sensitization or irritation is reported during use, the treatment should be discontinued.

Information for the Patient:

The patient should be cautioned against premature discontinuation of the medication during menstruation or in response to relief of symptoms.

Carcinogenesis:

Long-term studies in animals have not been performed to evaluate the carcinogenic potential of this drug.

Mutagenesis:

Butoconazole nitrate was not mutagenic when tested on microbial indicator organisms.

Impairment of Fertility:

No impairment of fertility was seen in rabbits or rats administered butoconazole nitrate in oral doses up to 30 mg/kg/day or 100 mg/kg/day respectively.

Pregnancy:

Pregnancy Category C: In pregnant rats administered 6 mg/kg/day (3-7 times the human dose) butoconazole nitrate intravaginally during the period of organogenesis, there was an increase in resorption rate and decrease in litter size, but no teratogenicity. Butoconazole nitrate had no apparent adverse effect when administered orally to pregnant rats throughout organogenesis, at dose levels up to 50 mg/kg/day. Daily oral doses of 100, 300, or 750 mg/kg resulted in fetal malformations (abdominal wall defects, cleft palate), but maternal stress was evident at these higher dose levels. There were no adverse effects on litters of rabbits receiving butoconazole nitrate orally, even at maternally stressful dose levels (e.g., 150 mg/kg). There are no adequate and well-controlled studies in pregnant women during the first trimester.

Butoconazole nitrate, like other azole antimycotic agents, causes dystocia in rats when treatment is extended through parturition. However, this effect was not apparent in rabbits treated with as much as 100 mg/kg orally.

In clinical studies, over 200 pregnant patients have used butoconazole nitrate cream 2% for 3 or 6 days during the second or third trimester and the drug had no adverse effect on the course of pregnancy. Follow-up reports available on infants born to these women reveal no adverse effects or complications that were attributable to the drug.

Nursing Mothers:

It is not known whether this drug is excreted in human milk. Because many drugs are excreted in human milk, caution should be exercised when butoconazole nitrate is administered to a nursing woman.

Pediatric Use:

Safety and effectiveness in children have not been established.

ADVERSE REACTIONS

Of the 561 patients treated with butoconazole nitrate cream 2% for 3 or 6 days in controlled clinical trials, 13 (2.3%) reported complaints probably related to therapy. Vulvar/vaginal burning occurred in 2.3%, vulvar itching in 0.9%, and discharge, soreness, swelling, and itching of the fingers each occurred in 0.2%. Nine patients (1.6%) discontinued because of these complaints.

DOSAGE AND ADMINISTRATION

Non-pregnant Patients: The recommended dose is one applicatorful of cream (approximately 5 grams) intravaginally at bedtime for three days. Treatment can be extended for an additional three days if necessary.

Pregnant Patients (2nd and 3rd trimesters only): The recommended dose is one applicatorful of cream (approximately 5 grams) intravaginally at bedtime for six days.

HOW SUPPLIED

FEMSTAT® PREFILL (butoconazole nitrate) Vaginal Cream 2% is available in cartons containing 3 single dose prefilled disposable applicators (NDC 0033-2280-16).

Store at room temperature. Avoid excessive heat, above 40°C (104°F), and avoid freezing.

CAUTION: Federal law prohibits dispensing without prescription.

U.S. Patent Nos. 4,078,071 and 4,636,202

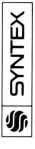

SYNTEX

SYNTEX LABORATORIES, INC.
PALO ALTO, CA 94304

02-2280-16-03

©March 1988

PHYSICIAN LABELING

BREVICON® 21-DAY Tablets
(norethindrone and ethinyl estradiol)

BREVICON® 28-DAY Tablets
(norethindrone and ethinyl estradiol)

NORINYL® 1 + 35 21-DAY Tablets
(norethindrone and ethinyl estradiol)

NORINYL® 1 + 35 28-DAY Tablets
(norethindrone and ethinyl estradiol)

NORINYL® 1 + 50 21-DAY Tablets
(norethindrone and mestranol)

NORINYL® 1 + 50 28-DAY Tablets
(norethindrone and mestranol)

NOR-QD® Tablets
(norethindrone)

The inactive orange tablets in the 28-day regimens of BREVICON, NORINYL 1 + 35 and NORINYL 1 + 50 contain the following ingredients: FD&C Yellow No. 6, lactose, magnesium stearate, povidone, and starch.

The yellow-green TRI-NORINYL tablets contain the following inactive ingredients: D&C Green No. 5, D&C Yellow No. 10, lactose, magnesium stearate, povidone, and starch.

The blue TRI-NORINYL tablets contain the following inactive ingredients: FD&C Blue No. 1, lactose, magnesium stearate, povidone, and starch.

The inactive orange tablets in the 28-day regimen contain the following inactive ingredients: FD&C Yellow No. 6, lactose, magnesium stearate, povidone, and starch.

CLINICAL PHARMACOLOGY

Combination oral contraceptives act by suppression of gonadotrophins. Although the primary mechanism of this action is inhibition of ovulation, other alterations include changes in the cervical mucus (which increase the difficulty of sperm entry into the uterus) and the endometrium (which may reduce the likelihood of implantation).

INDICATIONS AND USAGE

Oral contraceptives are indicated for the prevention of pregnancy in women who elect to use these products as a method of contraception.

Oral contraceptives are highly effective. Table I lists the typical accidental pregnancy rates for users of combination oral contraceptives and other methods of contraception.[1] The efficacy of these contraceptive methods, except sterilization, depends upon the reliability with which they are used. Correct and consistent use of methods can result in lower failure rates.

TRI-NORINYL® 21-DAY Tablets
(norethindrone and ethinyl estradiol)

TRI-NORINYL® 28-DAY Tablets
(norethindrone and ethinyl estradiol)

ORAL CONTRACEPTIVE AGENTS

DESCRIPTION

BREVICON 21-DAY Tablets provide an oral contraceptive regimen consisting of 21 blue tablets containing norethindrone 0.5 mg and ethinyl estradiol 0.035 mg.

BREVICON 28-DAY Tablets provide a continuous oral contraceptive regimen consisting of 21 blue tablets containing norethindrone 0.5 mg and ethinyl estradiol 0.035 mg and 7 orange tablets containing inert ingredients.

NORINYL 1 + 35 21-DAY Tablets provide an oral contraceptive regimen consisting of 21 yellow-green tablets containing norethindrone 1 mg and ethinyl estradiol 0.035 mg.

NORINYL 1 + 35 28-DAY Tablets provide a continuous oral contraceptive regimen consisting of 21 yellow-green tablets containing norethindrone 1 mg and ethinyl estradiol 0.035 mg followed by 7 orange tablets containing inert ingredients.

NORINYL 1 + 50 21-DAY Tablets provide an oral contraceptive regimen consisting of 21 white tablets containing norethindrone 1 mg and mestranol 0.05 mg.

NORINYL 1 + 50 28-DAY Tablets provide a continuous oral contraceptive regimen consisting of 21 white tablets containing norethindrone 1 mg and mestranol 0.05 mg and 7 orange tablets containing inert ingredients.

NOR-QD Tablets provide a continuous oral contraceptive regimen of one yellow norethindrone 0.35 mg tablet daily.

TRI-NORINYL 21-DAY Tablets provide an oral contraceptive regimen of 7 blue tablets followed by 9 yellow-green tablets and 5 more blue tablets. Each blue tablet contains norethindrone 0.5 mg and ethinyl estradiol 0.035 mg and each yellow-green tablet contains norethindrone 1 mg and ethinyl estradiol 0.035 mg.

TRI-NORINYL 28-DAY Tablets provide a continuous oral contraceptive regimen of 7 blue tablets, 9 yellow-green tablets, 5 more blue tablets, and then 7 orange tablets. Each blue tablet contains norethindrone 0.5 mg and ethinyl estradiol 0.035 mg, each yellow-green tablet contains norethindrone 1 mg and ethinyl estradiol 0.035 mg, and each orange tablet contains inert ingredients.

Norethindrone is a potent progestational agent with the chemical name 17-Hydroxy-19-nor-17α-pregn-4-en-20-yn-3-one. Ethinyl estradiol is an estrogen with the chemical name 19-nor-17α-pregna-1,3,5(10)-trien-20-yne-3,17-diol. Mestranol is an estrogen with the chemical name 3-Methoxy-19-nor-17α-pregna-1,3,5(10)-trien-20-yn-17-ol. Their structural formulae follow:

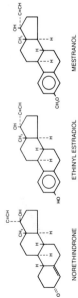

NORETHINDRONE

ETHINYL ESTRADIOL

MESTRANOL

The blue BREVICON tablets contain the following inactive ingredients: FD&C Blue No. 1, lactose, magnesium stearate, povidone, and starch.

The yellow-green NORINYL 1 + 35 tablets contain the following inactive ingredients: D&C Green No. 5, D&C Yellow No. 10, lactose, magnesium stearate, povidone, and starch.

The white NORINYL 1 + 50 tablets contain the following inactive ingredients: lactose, magnesium stearate, povidone, and starch.

The yellow NOR-QD tablets contain the following inactive ingredients: D&C yellow No. 10, FD&C Yellow No. 6, lactose, magnesium stearate, povidone, and starch.

TABLE I: LOWEST EXPECTED AND TYPICAL FAILURE RATES DURING THE FIRST YEAR OF CONTINUOUS USE OF A METHOD

% of Women Experiencing an Accidental Pregnancy in the First Year of Continuous Use

Method	Lowest Expected[a]	Typical[b]
(No Contraception)	(89)	(89)
Oral contraceptives		
combined	0.1	3
progestogen only	0.5	N/A[c]
Diaphragm with spermicidal cream or jelly	3	18
Spermicides alone (foam, creams, jellies and vaginal suppositories)	3	21
Vaginal Sponge		
Nulliparous	5	18
Multiparous	>8	>28
IUD (medicated)	1	6[d]
Condom without spermicides	2	12
Periodic abstinence (all methods)	2-10	20
Female sterilization	0.2	0.4
Male sterilization	0.1	0.15

Adapted from J. Trussell and K. Kost, Table 11[1]

[a] The authors' best guess of the percentage of women expected to experience an accidental pregnancy among couples who initiate a method (not necessarily for the first time) and who use it consistently and correctly during the first year if they do not stop for any other reason.

[b] This term represents "typical" couples who initiate use of a method (not necessarily for the first time), who experience an accidental pregnancy during the first year, if they do not stop use for any other reason. The authors derive these data largely from the National Surveys of Family Growth (NSFG), 1976 and 1982.

[c] N/A—Data not available from the NSFG, 1976 and 1982.

[d] Combined typical rate for both medicated and non-medicated IUD. The rate for medicated IUD alone is not available.

CONTRAINDICATIONS

Oral contraceptives should not be used in women who have the following conditions:

- Thrombophlebitis or thromboembolic disorders
- A past history of deep vein thrombophlebitis or thromboembolic disorders
- Cerebral vascular or coronary artery disease
- Known or suspected carcinoma of the breast
- Carcinoma of the endometrium, and known or suspected estrogen-dependent neoplasia
- Undiagnosed abnormal genital bleeding
- Cholestatic jaundice of pregnancy or jaundice with prior pill use
- Hepatic adenomas, carcinomas or benign liver tumors
- Known or suspected pregnancy

WARNINGS

Cigarette smoking increases the risk of serious cardiovascular side effects from oral contraceptive use. This risk increases with age and with heavy smoking (15 or more cigarettes per day) and is quite marked in women over 35 years of age. Women who use oral contraceptives should be strongly advised not to smoke.

The use of oral contraceptives is associated with increased risks of several serious conditions including myocardial infarction, thromboembolism, stroke, hepatic neoplasia and gallbladder disease, although the risk of serious morbidity and mortality increases significantly in the presence of other underlying risk factors such as hypertension, hyperlipidemias, hypercholesterolemia, obesity and diabetes.[2-5]

Practitioners prescribing oral contraceptives should be familiar with the following information relating to these risks.

The information contained in this package insert is principally based on studies carried out in patients who used oral contraceptives with formulations containing 0.05 mg or higher of estrogen.[6,11] The effects of long-term use with lower dose formulations of both estrogens and progestogens remain to be determined.

Throughout this labeling, epidemiological studies reported are of two types: retrospective or case control studies and prospective or cohort studies. Case control studies provide a measure of the relative risk of disease. Relative risk, the *ratio* of the incidence of a disease among oral contraceptive users to that among non-users, cannot be assessed directly from case control studies, but the odds ratio obtained is a measure of relative risk. The relative risk does not provide information on the actual clinical occurrence of a disease. Cohort studies provide not only a measure of the relative risk but a measure of attributable risk, which is the *difference* in the incidence of disease between oral contraceptive users and non-users. The attributable risk does provide information about the actual occurrence of a disease in the population.[12,13]

1. THROMBOEMBOLIC DISORDERS AND OTHER VASCULAR PROBLEMS

a. Myocardial Infarction

An increased risk of myocardial infarction has been attributed to oral contraceptive use. This risk is primarily in smokers or women with other underlying risk factors for coronary artery disease such as hypertension, hypercholesterolemia, morbid obesity and diabetes.[2,5,13] The relative risk of heart attack for current oral contraceptive users has been estimated to be 2 to 6.[2,14-19] The risk is very low under the age of 30. However, there is the possibility of a risk of cardiovascular disease even in very young women who take oral contraceptives.

Smoking in combination with oral contraceptive use has been shown to contribute substantially to the incidence of myocardial infarctions in women 35 or older, with smoking accounting for the majority of excess cases.[20]

Mortality rates associated with circulatory disease have been shown to increase substantially in smokers over the age of 35 and non-smokers over the age of 40 among women who use oral contraceptives (see Table II).[16]

TABLE II: CIRCULATORY DISEASE MORTALITY RATES PER 100,000 WOMAN YEARS BY AGE, SMOKING STATUS AND ORAL CONTRACEPTIVE USE

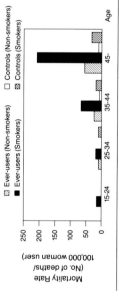

Adapted from P.M. Layde and V. Beral, Table V[16]

Oral contraceptives may compound the effects of well-known risk factors for coronary artery disease, such as hypertension, diabetes, hyperlipidemias, hypercholesterolemia, age and obesity.[3,13,21] In particular, some progestogens are known to decrease HDL cholesterol and impair oral glucose tolerance, while estrogens may create a state of hyperinsulinism.[21,25] Oral contraceptives have been shown to increase blood pressure among users (see WARNINGS, section 9). Similar effects on risk factors have been associated with an increased risk of heart disease. Oral contraceptives must be used with caution in women with cardiovascular disease risk factors.

b. Thromboembolism

An increased risk of thromboembolic and thrombotic disease associated with the use of oral contraceptives is well established. Case control studies have found the relative risk of users compared to non-users to be 3 for the first episode of superficial venous thrombosis, 4 to 11 for deep vein thrombosis or pulmonary embolism, and 1.5 to 6 for women with predisposing conditions for venous thromboembolic disease.[12,13,26-31] One cohort study has shown the relative risk to be somewhat lower, about 3 for new

Because of these changes in practice and, also, because of some limited new data which suggest that the risk of cardiovascular disease with the use of oral contraceptives may now be less than previously observed,[78,79] the Fertility and Maternal Health Drugs Advisory Committee was asked to review the topic in 1989. The Committee concluded that although cardiovascular disease risks may be increased with oral contraceptive use after age 40 in healthy non-smoking women (even with the newer low-dose formulations), there are greater potential health risks associated with pregnancy in older women and with the alternative surgical and medical procedures which may be necessary if such women do not have access to effective and acceptable means of contraception.

Therefore, the Committee recommended that the benefits of oral contraceptive use by healthy non-smoking women over 40 may outweigh the possible risks. Of course, older women, as all women who take oral contraceptives, should take the lowest possible dose formulation that is effective.[80]

TABLE III: ESTIMATED ANNUAL NUMBER OF BIRTH-RELATED OR METHOD-RELATED DEATHS ASSOCIATED WITH CONTROL OF FERTILITY PER 100,000 NONSTERILE WOMEN, BY FERTILITY CONTROL METHOD ACCORDING TO AGE

Method of control and outcome	15-19	20-24	25-29	30-34	35-39	40-44
No fertility control methods*	7.0	7.4	9.1	14.8	25.7	28.2
Oral contraceptives non-smoker**	0.3	0.5	0.9	1.9	13.8	31.6
Oral contraceptives smoker**	2.2	3.4	6.6	13.5	51.1	117.2
IUD**	0.8	0.8	1.0	1.0	1.4	1.4
Condom*	1.1	1.6	0.7	0.2	0.3	0.4
Diaphragm/Spermicide*	1.9	1.2	1.2	1.3	2.2	2.8
Periodic abstinence*	2.5	1.6	1.6	1.7	2.9	3.6

*Deaths are birth-related
**Deaths are method-related

Estimates adapted from H.W. Ory, Table 3[41]

3. CARCINOMA OF THE BREAST AND REPRODUCTIVE ORGANS

Numerous epidemiological studies have been performed on the incidence of breast, endometrial, ovarian and cervical cancer in women using oral contraceptives. The evidence in the literature suggests that use of oral contraceptives is not associated with an increase in the risk of developing breast cancer, regardless of the age and parity of first use or with most of the marketed brands and doses.[42,43] The Cancer and Steroid Hormone study also showed no latent effect on the risk of breast cancer for at least a decade following long-term use.[43] A few studies have shown a slightly increased relative risk of developing breast cancer,[44,47] although the methodology of these studies, which included differences in examination of users and non-users and differences in age at start of use, has been questioned.[47-49] Some studies have reported an increased relative risk of developing breast cancer, particularly at a younger age. This increased relative risk appears to be related to duration of use.[81,82]

Some studies suggest that oral contraceptive use has been associated with an increase in the risk of cervical intraepithelial neoplasia in some populations of women.[50-53] However, there continues to be controversy about the extent to which such findings may be due to differences in sexual behavior and other factors.

In spite of many studies of the relationship between oral contraceptive use and breast or cervical cancers, a cause and effect relationship has not been established.

4. HEPATIC NEOPLASIA

Benign hepatic adenomas are associated with oral contraceptive use although the incidence of benign tumors is rare in the United States. Indirect calculations have estimated the attributable risk to be in the range of 3.3 cases per 100,000 for users, a risk that increases after 4 or more years of use.[54] Rupture of rare, benign, hepatic adenomas may cause death through intra-abdominal hemorrhage.[55,56]

Studies in the United States and Britain have shown an increased risk of developing hepatocellular carcinoma in long-term (>8 years) oral contraceptive users.[57,59] However, these cancers are extremely rare in the United States and the attributable risk (the excess incidence) of liver cancers in oral contraceptive users is less than 1 per 1,000,000 users.

5. OCULAR LESIONS

There have been clinical case reports of retinal thrombosis associated with the use of oral contraceptives. Oral contraceptives should be discontinued if there is unexplained partial or complete loss of vision; onset of proptosis or diplopia; papilledema; or retinal vascular lesions. Appropriate diagnostic and therapeutic measures should be undertaken immediately.

6. ORAL CONTRACEPTIVE USE BEFORE OR DURING EARLY PREGNANCY

Extensive epidemiological studies have revealed no increased risk of birth defects in women who have used oral contraceptives prior to pregnancy.[60-62] More recent studies do not suggest a teratogenic effect, particularly insofar as cardiac anomalies and limb reduction defects are concerned, when taken inadvertently during early pregnancy.[60, 61, 63, 64]

The administration of oral contraceptives to induce withdrawal bleeding should not be used as a test for pregnancy. Oral contraceptives should not be used during pregnancy to treat threatened or habitual abortion.

It is recommended that for any patient who has missed 2 consecutive period..., pregnancy should be ruled out before continuing oral contraceptive use. If the patient has not adhered to the prescribed schedule, the possibility of pregnancy should be considered at the time of the first missed period. Oral contraceptive use should be discontinued if pregnancy is confirmed.

7. GALLBLADDER DISEASE

Earlier studies have reported an increased lifetime relative risk of gallbladder surgery in users of oral contraceptives and estrogens.[65-66] More recent studies, however, have shown that the relative risk of developing gallbladder disease among oral contraceptive users may be minimal.[67] The recent findings of minimal risk may be related to the use of oral contraceptive formulations containing lower hormonal doses of estrogens and progestogens.[68]

8. CARBOHYDRATE AND LIPID METABOLIC EFFECTS

Oral contraceptives have been shown to impair oral glucose tolerance.[69] Oral contraceptives containing greater than 0.075 mg of estrogen cause glucose intolerance with impaired insulin secretion, while lower doses of estrogen may produce less glucose intolerance.[70] Progestogens increase insulin secretion and create insulin resistance, this effect varying with different progestational agents.[25, 71] However, in the non-diabetic woman, oral contraceptives appear to have no effect on fasting blood glucose.[69] Because of these demonstrated effects, prediabetic and diabetic women should be carefully observed while taking oral contraceptives.

Some women may develop persistent hypertriglyceridemia while on the pill.[72] As discussed earlier (see WARNINGS, sections 1a. and 1d.), changes in serum triglycerides and lipoprotein levels have been reported in oral contraceptive users.[23]

9. ELEVATED BLOOD PRESSURE

An increase in blood pressure has been reported in women taking oral contraceptives. The incidence of risk also was reported to increase with continued use and among older women.[66] Data from the Royal College of General Practitioners and subsequent randomized trials have shown that the incidence of hypertension increases with increasing concentrations of progestogens.

Women with a history of hypertension or hypertension-related diseases or renal disease should be encouraged to use another method of contraception. If women elect to use oral contraceptives, they should be monitored closely and if significant elevation of blood pressure occurs oral contraceptives should be discontinued. For most women, elevated blood pressure will return to normal after stopping oral contraceptives and there is no difference in the occurrence of hypertension among ever- and never-users.[73-75]

10. HEADACHE

The onset or exacerbation of migraine or development of headache with a new pattern which is recurrent, persistent or severe requires discontinuation of oral contraceptives and evaluation of the cause.

11. BLEEDING IRREGULARITIES

Breakthrough bleeding and spotting are sometimes encountered in patients on oral contraceptives, especially during the first 3 months of use. Non-hormonal causes should be considered and adequate diagnostic measures taken to rule out malignancy or pregnancy in the event of breakthrough bleeding, as in the case of any abnormal vaginal bleeding. If pathology has been excluded, time or a change to another formula-

cases (subjects with no past history of venous thrombosis or varicose veins) and about 4.5 for new cases requiring hospitalization.[32] The risk of thromboembolic disease due to oral contraceptives is not related to length of use and disappears after pill use is stopped.[12]

A 2- to 6-fold increase in relative risk of post-operative thromboembolic complications has been reported with the use of oral contraceptives.[18] If feasible, oral contraceptives should be discontinued at least 4 weeks prior to and for 2 weeks after elective surgery and during and following prolonged immobilization. Since the immediate postpartum period also is associated with an increased risk of thromboembolism, oral contraceptives should be started no earlier than 4 to 6 weeks after delivery in women who elect not to breast feed.[33]

c. Cerebrovascular diseases

An increase in both the relative and attributable risks of cerebrovascular events (thrombotic and hemorrhagic strokes) has been shown in users of oral contraceptives. In general, the risk is greatest among older (>35 years), hypertensive women who also smoke. Hypertension was found to be a risk factor for both users and non-users for both types of strokes while smoking interacted to increase the risk for hemorrhagic strokes.[34]

In a large study, the relative risk of thrombotic strokes has been shown to range from 3 for normotensive users to 14 for users with severe hypertension.[35] The relative risk of hemorrhagic stroke is reported to be 1.2 for non-smokers who used oral contraceptives, 2.6 for smokers who did not use oral contraceptives, 7.6 for smokers who used oral contraceptives, 1.8 for normotensive users and 25.7 for users with severe hypertension.[35] The attributable risk also is greater in women 35 or older and among smokers.[13]

d. Dose-related risk of vascular disease from oral contraceptives

A positive association has been observed between the amount of estrogen and progestogen in oral contraceptives and the risk of vascular disease.[36-38] A decline in serum high density lipoproteins (HDL) has been reported with some progestational agents.[22,24] A decline in serum high density lipoproteins has been associated with an increased incidence of ischemic heart disease.[39] Because estrogens increase HDL cholesterol, the net effect of an oral contraceptive depends on a balance achieved between doses of estrogen and progestogen and the nature and absolute amount of progestogens used in the contraceptives. The amount of both hormones should be considered in the choice of an oral contraceptive.[37]

Minimizing exposure to estrogen and progestogen is in keeping with good principles of therapeutics. For any particular estrogen/progestogen combination, the dosage regimen prescribed should be one which contains the least amount of estrogen and progestogen that is compatible with a low failure rate and the needs of the individual patient. New acceptors of oral contraceptive agents should be started on preparations containing the lowest estrogen content that produces satisfactory results for the individual.

e. Persistence of risk of vascular disease

There are three studies which have shown persistence of risk of vascular disease for ever-users of oral contraceptives.[17, 34, 40] In a study in the United States, the risk of developing myocardial infarction after discontinuing oral contraceptives persists for at least 9 years for women 40-49 years who had used oral contraceptives for 5 or more years, but this increased risk was not demonstrated in other age groups.[17] In another study in Great Britain, the risk of developing cerebrovascular disease persisted for at least 6 years after discontinuation of oral contraceptives, although excess risk was very small.[40] Subarachnoid hemorrhage also has a significantly increased relative risk after termination of use of oral contraceptives.[34] However, these studies were performed with oral contraceptive formulations containing 0.05 mg or higher of estrogen.

2. ESTIMATES OF MORTALITY FROM CONTRACEPTIVE USE

One study gathered data from a variety of sources which have estimated the mortality rates associated with different methods of contraception at different ages (see Table III).[41] These estimates include the combined risk of death associated with contraceptive methods plus the risk attributable to pregnancy in the event of method failure. Each method of contraception has its specific benefits and risks. The study concluded that with the exception of oral contraceptive users 35 and older who smoke and 40 and older who do not smoke, mortality associated with all methods of birth control is low and below that associated with childbirth. The observation of a possible increase in risk of mortality with age for oral contraceptive users is based on data gathered in the 1970's—but not reported in the U.S. until 1983.[16, 41] However, current clinical practice involves the use of lower estrogen dose formulations combined with careful restriction of oral contraceptive use to women who do not have the various risk factors listed in this labeling.

tion may solve the problem. In the event of amenorrhea, pregnancy should be ruled out.

Some women may encounter post-pill amenorrhea or oligomenorrhea, especially when such a condition was pre-existent.

PRECAUTIONS

1. PHYSICAL EXAMINATION AND FOLLOW-UP

A complete medical history and physical examination should be taken prior to the initiation of oral contraceptives and at least annually during use of oral contraceptives. These physical examinations should include special reference to blood pressure, breasts, abdomen and pelvic organs, including cervical cytology and relevant laboratory tests. In case of undiagnosed, persistent or recurrent abnormal vaginal bleeding, appropriate diagnostic measures should be conducted to rule out malignancy. Women with a strong family history of breast cancer or who have breast nodules should be monitored with particular care.

2. LIPID DISORDERS

Women who are being treated for hyperlipidemias should be followed closely if they elect to use oral contraceptives. Some progestogens may elevate LDL levels and may render the control of hyperlipidemias more difficult.

3. LIVER FUNCTION

If jaundice develops in any woman receiving oral contraceptives the medication should be discontinued. Steroid hormones may be poorly metabolized in patients with impaired liver function.

4. FLUID RETENTION

Oral contraceptives may cause some degree of fluid retention. They should be prescribed with caution, and only with careful monitoring, in patients with conditions which might be aggravated by fluid retention.

5. EMOTIONAL DISORDERS

Women with a history of depression should be carefully observed and the drug discontinued if depression recurs to a serious degree.

6. CONTACT LENSES

Contact lens wearers who develop visual changes or changes in lens tolerance should be assessed by an ophthalmologist.

7. DRUG INTERACTIONS

Reduced efficacy and increased incidence of breakthrough bleeding and menstrual irregularities have been associated with concomitant use of rifampin. A similar association though less marked, has been suggested with barbiturates, phenylbutazone, phenytoin sodium, and possibly with griseofulvin, ampicillin and tetracyclines.[76]

8. INTERACTIONS WITH LABORATORY TESTS

Certain endocrine and liver function tests and blood components may be affected by oral contraceptives:

a. Increased prothrombin and factors VII, VIII, IX, and X; decreased antithrombin 3; increased norepinephrine-induced platelet aggregability.

b. Increased thyroid binding globulin (TBG) leading to increased circulating total thyroid hormone, as measured by protein-bound iodine (PBI), T4 by column or by radioimmunoassay. Free T3 resin uptake is decreased, reflecting the elevated TBG. Free T4 concentration is unaltered.

c. Other binding proteins may be elevated in serum.

d. Sex steroid binding globulins are increased and result in elevated levels of total circulating sex steroids and corticoids; however, free or biologically active levels remain unchanged.

e. Triglycerides may be increased.

f. Glucose tolerance may be decreased.

g. Serum folate levels may be depressed by oral contraceptive therapy. This may be of clinical significance if a woman becomes pregnant shortly after discontinuing oral contraceptives.

9. CARCINOGENESIS

See **WARNINGS** section.

10. PREGNANCY

Pregnancy Category X. See **CONTRAINDICATIONS** and **WARNINGS** sections.

Effects on menses:
- Increased menstrual cycle regularity
- Decreased blood loss and decreased incidence of iron deficiency anemia
- Decreased incidence of dysmenorrhea

Effects related to inhibition of ovulation:
- Decreased incidence of functional ovarian cysts
- Decreased incidence of ectopic pregnancies

Effects from long-term use:
- Decreased incidence of fibroadenomas and fibrocystic disease of the breast
- Decreased incidence of acute pelvic inflammatory disease
- Decreased incidence of endometrial cancer
- Decreased incidence of ovarian cancer

DOSAGE AND ADMINISTRATION

To achieve maximum contraceptive effectiveness, oral contraceptives must be taken exactly as described and at intervals not exceeding 24 hours.

BREVICON, NORINYL 1 + 35, NORINYL 1 + 50

21-Day Schedule: For the initial cycle of therapy the first tablet may be taken on Day 5 of the menstrual cycle, counting the first day of menstrual flow as Day 1 (DAY 5 START), or the first tablet may be taken on the first Sunday after menstrual flow begins (SUNDAY START). For SUNDAY START when menstrual flow begins on Sunday, the first tablet is taken on that day. With either DAY 5 START or SUNDAY START, 1 tablet is taken each day at the same time for 21 days. No tablets are taken for 7 days, then, whether bleeding has stopped or not, a new course is started of 1 tablet a day for 21 days. This institutes a 3 weeks on, 1 week off dosage regimen.

28-Day Schedule: For the initial cycle of therapy the first tablet may be taken on Day 5 of the menstrual cycle, counting the first day of menstrual flow as Day 1 (DAY 5 START), or the first tablet may be taken on the first Sunday after menstrual flow begins (SUNDAY START). For SUNDAY START when menstrual flow begins on Sunday, the first tablet is taken on that day. With either DAY 5 START or SUNDAY START, 1 white, yellow-green, or blue tablet is taken each day at the same time for 21 days. Then the orange tablets are taken, 1 each evening at bedtime for 7 days. After all 28 tablets have been taken, whether bleeding has stopped or not, repeat the same dosage schedule beginning on the following day.

NOR-QD (norethindrone) is administered as a continuous daily dosage regimen starting on the first day of menstruation, i.e., 1 tablet each day, every day. Tablets should be taken at the same time each day and continued daily, without interruption, whether bleeding occurs or not. This is especially important for patients new to progestogen-only oral contraception. The patient should be advised that if prolonged bleeding occurs, she should consult her physician.

TRI-NORINYL

21-Day Regimen Dosage Schedule: The first blue tablet is taken on the first Sunday after menstrual flow begins. If menstrual flow begins on Sunday, the first blue tablet is taken on that day. One blue tablet is taken each evening at bedtime for 7 days, then one yellow-green tablet each evening for 9 days, then one blue tablet each evening for 5 days. No tablets are taken for 7 days; then, whether bleeding has stopped or not, a new sequence of tablets is started for 21 days. This institutes a three weeks on, one week off dosage regimen.

28-Day Regimen Dosage Schedule: The first blue tablet is taken on the first Sunday after menstrual flow begins. If menstrual flow begins on Sunday, the first blue tablet is taken on that day. One blue tablet is taken each evening at bedtime for 7 days, then one yellow-green tablet each evening for 9 days, then one blue tablet each evening for 5 days, then one orange (inert) tablet each evening for 7 days. After all 28 tablets have been taken, whether bleeding has stopped or not, the same dosage schedule is repeated beginning on the following day.

INSTRUCTIONS TO PATIENTS

- To achieve maximum contraceptive effectiveness, the oral contraceptive pill must be taken exactly as directed and at intervals not exceeding 24 hours.
- Important: Women should be instructed to use an additional method of protection until after the first 7 days of administration *in the initial cycle.*
- Due to the normally increased risk of thromboembolism occurring postpartum, women should be instructed not to initiate treatment with oral contraceptives earlier than 4 weeks after a full-term delivery. If pregnancy is terminated in the first 12 weeks, the patient should be instructed to start oral contraceptives immediately or within 7 days. If pregnancy is terminated after 12 weeks, the patient should be instructed to start oral contraceptives after 2 weeks.[33,77]
- If spotting or breakthrough bleeding should occur, the patient should continue the

11. NURSING MOTHERS

Small amounts of oral contraceptive steroids have been identified in the milk of nursing mothers and a few adverse effects on the child have been reported, including jaundice and breast enlargement. In addition, oral contraceptives given in the postpartum period may interfere with lactation by decreasing the quantity and quality of breast milk. If possible, the nursing mother should be advised not to use oral contraceptives but to use other forms of contraception until she has completely weaned her child.

INFORMATION FOR THE PATIENT

See **PATIENT LABELING.**

ADVERSE REACTIONS

An increased risk of the following serious adverse reactions has been associated with the use of oral contraceptives (see **WARNINGS** section):

- Thrombophlebitis
- Arterial thromboembolism
- Pulmonary embolism
- Myocardial infarction
- Cerebral hemorrhage
- Cerebral thrombosis
- Hypertension
- Gallbladder disease
- Hepatic adenomas, carcinomas or benign liver tumors

There is evidence of an association between the following conditions and the use of oral contraceptives, although additional confirmatory studies are needed:

- Mesenteric thrombosis
- Retinal thrombosis

The following adverse reactions have been reported in patients receiving oral contraceptives and are believed to be drug-related:

- Nausea
- Vomiting
- Gastrointestinal symptoms (such as abdominal cramps and bloating)
- Breakthrough bleeding
- Spotting
- Change in menstrual flow
- Amenorrhea
- Temporary infertility after discontinuation of treatment
- Edema
- Melasma which may persist
- Breast changes: tenderness, enlargement, secretion
- Change in weight (increase or decrease)
- Change in cervical erosion and secretion
- Diminution in lactation when given immediately postpartum
- Cholestatic jaundice
- Migraine
- Rash (allergic)
- Mental depression
- Reduced tolerance to carbohydrates
- Vaginal candidiasis
- Change in corneal curvature (steepening)
- Intolerance to contact lenses

The following adverse reactions have been reported in users of oral contraceptives and the association has been neither confirmed nor refuted:

- Pre-menstrual syndrome
- Cataracts
- Changes in appetite
- Cystitis-like syndrome
- Headache
- Nervousness
- Dizziness
- Hirsutism
- Loss of scalp hair
- Erythema multiforme
- Erythema nodosum
- Hemorrhagic eruption
- Vaginitis
- Porphyria
- Impaired renal function
- Hemolytic uremic syndrome
- Budd-Chiari syndrome
- Acne
- Changes in libido
- Colitis

OVERDOSAGE

Serious ill effects have not been reported following acute ingestion of large doses of oral contraceptives by young children. Overdosage may cause nausea, and withdrawal bleeding may occur in females.

NON-CONTRACEPTIVE HEALTH BENEFITS

The following non-contraceptive health benefits related to the use of oral contraceptives are supported by epidemiological studies which largely utilized oral contraceptive formulations containing estrogen doses exceeding 0.035 mg of ethinyl estradiol or 0.05 mg of mestranol.[6-11]

---

medication according to the schedule. Should spotting or breakthrough bleeding persist, the patient should notify her physician.

- If the patient misses 1 pill, she should be instructed to take it as soon as she remembers and then take the next pill at the regular time. If the patient has missed 2 pills, she should take 1 of the missed pills as soon as she remembers and discard the other missed pill. She should then take her next pill at the regular time. Furthermore, she should use an additional method of contraception in addition to taking her pills for the remainder of the cycle.
- If the patient has missed more than 2 pills, she should be instructed to discontinue taking the remaining pills and to use an alternative method of contraception until pregnancy has been ruled out.
- Use of oral contraceptives in the event of a missed menstrual period:
  1. If the patient has not adhered to the prescribed dosage regimen, the possibility of pregnancy should be considered after the first missed period and oral contraceptives should be withheld until pregnancy has been ruled out.
  2. If the patient has adhered to the prescribed regimen and misses 2 consecutive periods, pregnancy should be ruled out before continuing the contraceptive regimen.

HOW SUPPLIED

BREVICON® 21-DAY Tablets and BREVICON® 28-DAY Tablets (norethindrone and ethinyl estradiol), and NORINYL® 1 + 35 21-DAY Tablets and NORINYL® 1 + 35 28-DAY Tablets (norethindrone and ethinyl estradiol), and NORINYL® 1 + 50 21-DAY Tablets and NORINYL® 1 + 50 28-DAY Tablets (norethindrone and mestranol) are available in 21-pill or 28-pill blister cards with a WALLETTE® pill dispenser. Each 28-pill card contains 7 orange inert pills.

NOR-QD® (norethindrone) tablets are available in 42-tablet dispensers.

TRI-NORINYL® 21-DAY Tablets and TRI-NORINYL® 28-DAY Tablets (norethindrone and ethinyl estradiol) are available in 21-pill or 28-pill blister cards with a WALLETTE® pill dispenser. Each 28-pill card contains 7 orange inert pills.

CAUTION: Federal law prohibits dispensing without prescription.

REFERENCES

1. Trussell, J., et al.: *Stud Fam Plann* 18(5):237–283, 1987. 2. Mann, J., et al.: *Br Med J* 2(5956):241–245, 1975. 3. Knopp, R.H.: *J Reprod Med* 31(9):913–921, 1986. 4. Mann, J.I. et al.: *Br Med J* 2:445–447, 1976. 5. Ory, H.: *JAMA* 237:2619–2622, 1977. 6. The Cancer and Steroid Hormone Study of the Centers for Disease Control: *JAMA* 249(2):1596–1599, 1983. 7. The Cancer and Steroid Hormone Study of the Centers for Disease Control: *JAMA* 257(6):796–800, 1987. 8. Ory, H.W.: *JAMA* 228(1):68–69, 1974. 9. Ory, H.W. et al.: *N Engl J Med* 294:419–422, 1976. 10. Ory, H.W.: *Fam Plann Perspect* 14:182–184, 1982. 11. Ory, H.W. et al.: *Making Choices*, New York, The Alan Guttmacher Institute, 1983. 12. Stadel, B.: *N Engl J Med* 305(11):612–618, 1981. 13. Stadel, B.: *N Engl J Med* 305(12):672–677, 1981. 14. Adam, S., et al.: *Br J Obstet Gynaecol* 88:838–845, 1981. 15. Mann, J., et al.: *Br Med J* 2(5965):245–248, 1975. 16. Royal College of General Practitioners' Oral Contraceptive Study: *Lancet* 1:541–546, 1981. 17. Slone, D., et al.: *N Engl J Med* 305(8):420–424, 1981. 18. Vessey, M.P.: *Br J Fam Plann* 6 (supplement): 1–12, 1980. 19. Russell-Briefel, R., et al.: *Prev Med* 15:352–362, 1986. 20. Goldbaum, G., et al.: *JAMA* 258(10):1339–1342, 1987. 21. LaRosa, J.C.: *J Reprod Med* 31(9):906–912, 1986. 22. Krauss, R.M., et al.: *Am J Obstet Gynecol* 145:446–452, 1983. 23. Wahl, P., et al.: *N Engl J Med* 308(15):862–867, 1983. 24. Wynn, V., et al.: *Am J Obstet Gynecol* 142(6):766–771, 1982. 25. Wynn, V., et al.: *J Reprod Med* 31(9):892–897, 1986. 26. Inman, W.H., et al.: *Br Med J* 2(5599):193–199, 1968. 27. Maguire, M.G., et al.: *Am J Epidemiol* 110(2):188–195, 1979. 28. Petitti, D., et al.: *JAMA* 242(11):1150–1154, 1979. 29. Vessey, M.P., et al.: *Br Med J* 2(5599):199–205, 1968. 30. Vessey, M.P., et al.: *Br Med J* 2(5668):651–657, 1969. 31. Porter, J.B., et al.: *Obstet Gynecol* 59(3):299–302, 1982. 32. Vessey, M.P., et al.: *J Biosoc Sci* 8:373–427, 1976. 33. Mishell, D.R., et al.: *Reproductive Endocrinology*, Philadelphia, F.A. Davis Co., 1979. 34. Petitti, D.B., et al.: *Lancet* 2:234–236, 1978. 35. Collaborative Group for the Study of Stroke in Young Women: *JAMA* 231(7):718–722, 1975. 36. Inman, W.H., et al.: *Br Med J* 2:203–209, 1970. 37. Meade, T.W., et al.: *Br Med J* 280(6224):1157–1161, 1980. 38. Kay, C.R.: *Am J Obstet Gynecol* 142(6):762–765, 1982. 39. Gordon, T., et al.: *Am J Med* 62:707–714, 1977. 40. Royal College of General Practitioners' Oral Contraception Study: *J Coll Gen Pract* 33:75–82, 1983. 41. Ory, H.W.: *Fam Plann Perspect* 15(2):57–63, 1983. 42. Paul, C., et al.: *Br Med J* 293:723–725, 1986. 43. The Cancer and Steroid Hormone Study of the Centers for Disease Control: *N Engl J Med* 315(7):405–411, 1986. 44. Pike, M.C., et al.: *Lancet* 2:926–929, 1983. 45. Miller, D.R., et al.: *Obstet Gynecol* 68:863–868, 1986. 46. Olsson, H., et al.: *Lancet* 2:748–749, 1985. 47. McPherson, K., et al.: *Br J Cancer* 56:653–660, 1987. 48. Huggins, G.R., et al.: *Fertil Steril* 47(5):733–761, 1987. 49. McPherson, K., et al.: *Br Med J* 293:709–710, 1986. 50. Ory, H., et al.: *Am J Obstet Gynecol* 124(6):573–577, 1976. 51. Vessey, M.P., et al.: *Lancet* 2:930, 1983. 52. Brinton, L.A., et al.: *Int J Cancer* 38:339–344, 1986. 53. WHO Collaborative Study of Neoplasia and Steroid Contraceptives: *B-*

Med. J. 290:961–965, 1985. **54.** Rooks, J.B., et al.: JAMA 242(7):644–648, 1979. **55.** Bein, N.N., et al.: Br J Surg 64:433–435, 1977. **56.** Klatskin, G.: Gastroenterology 73:386–394, 1977. **57.** Henderson, B.E., et al.: Br J Cancer 48:437–440, 1983. **58.** Neuberger, J., et al.: Br Med J 292:1355–1357, 1986. **59.** Forman, D., et al.: Br Med J 292:1357–1361, 1986. **60.** Harlap, S., et al.: Obstet Gynecol 55(4):447–452, 1980. **61.** Savolainen, E., et al.: Am J Obstet Gynecol 140(5):521–524, 1981. **62.** Janerich, D.T., et al.: Am J Epidemiol 112(1):73–79, 1980. **63.** Ferencz, C., et al.: Teratology 21:225–239, 1980. **64.** Rothman, K.J., et al.: Am J Epidemiol 109(4):433–439, 1979. **65.** Boston Collaborative Drug Surveillance Program: Lancet 1:1399–1404, 1973. **66.** Royal College of General Practitioners: Oral contraceptives and health. New York, Pittman, 1974. **67.** Rome Group for the Epidemiology and Prevention of Cholelithiasis: Am J Epidemiol 119(5):796–805, 1984. **68.** Strom, B.L., et al.: Clin Pharmacol Ther 39(3):335–341, 1986. **69.** Perlman, J.A., et al.: J Chronic Dis 38(10):857–864, 1985. **70.** Wynn, V., et al.: Lancet 1:1045–1049, 1979. **71.** Wynn, V.: Progesterone and Progestin, New York, Raven Press, 1983. **72.** Wynn, V., et al.: Lancet 2:720–723, 1966. **73.** Fisch, I.R., et al.: JAMA 237(23):2499–2503, 1977. **74.** Laragh, J.H.: Am J Obstet Gynecol 126(1):141–147, 1976. **75.** Ramcharan, S., et al.: Pharmacology of Steroid Contraceptive Drugs, New York, Raven Press, 1977. **76.** Stockley, I.: Pharm 216:140–143, 1976. **77.** Dickey, R.P.: Managing Contraceptive Pill Patients, Oklahoma, Creative Infomatics Inc., 1984. **78.** Porter, J.B., Hunter, J., Jick H., et al.: Obstet Gynecol 1985;66:1–4. **79.** Porter J.B., Hershel J., Walker A.M.: Obstet Gynecol 1987;70:29–32. **80.** Fertility and Maternal Health Drugs Advisory Committee, F.D.A., October, 1989. **81.** Schlesselman J., Stadel B.V., Murray P., Lai S.: Breast cancer in relation to early use of oral contraceptives. JAMA 1988;259:1828–1833. **82.** Hennekens C.H., Speizer F.E., Lipnick R.J., Rosner B., Bain C., Belanger C., Stampfer M.J., Willett W., Peto R.: A case-control study of oral contraceptive use and breast cancer. JNCl 1984:72:39–42.

DETAILED PATIENT LABELING

INTRODUCTION

Any woman who considers using oral contraceptives ("birth control pills" or "the pill") should understand the benefits and risks of using this form of birth control. This leaflet will give you much of the information you will need to make this decision and also will help you determine if you are at risk of developing any of the serious side effects of the pill. It will tell you how to use the pill properly so that it will be as effective as possible. However, this leaflet is not a replacement for a careful discussion between you and your health care provider. You should discuss the information provided in this leaflet with him or her, both when you first start taking the pill and during your regular visits. You also should follow the advice of your health care provider with regard to regular check-ups while you are on the pill.

EFFECTIVENESS OF ORAL CONTRACEPTIVES

Oral contraceptives are used to prevent pregnancy and are more effective than other non-surgical methods of birth control. When they are taken correctly, without missing any pills, the chance of becoming pregnant is less than 1% (1 pregnancy per 100 women per year of use). Typical failure rates are actually 3% per year. The chance of becoming pregnant increases with each missed pill during a menstrual cycle.

In comparison, typical failure rates for other non-surgical methods of birth control during the first year are as follows:

IUD: 6%
Diaphragm with spermicides: 18%
Spermicides alone: 21%
Vaginal sponge: 18 to 30%
Condom alone: 12%
Periodic abstinence: 20%
No methods: 89%

WHO SHOULD NOT TAKE ORAL CONTRACEPTIVES

Cigarette smoking increases the risk of serious cardiovascular side effects from oral contraceptive use. This risk increases with age and with heavy smoking (15 or more cigarettes per day) and is quite marked in women over 35 years of age. Women who use oral contraceptives are strongly advised not to smoke.

Some women should not use the pill. For example, you should not take the pill if you are pregnant or think you may be pregnant. You also should not use the pill if you have any of the following conditions:

- A history of heart attack or stroke
- Blood clots in the legs (thrombophlebitis), brain (stroke), lungs (pulmonary embo-

---

5. Cancer of the breast and reproductive organs

There is, at present, no confirmed evidence that oral contraceptives increase the risk of cancer of the reproductive organs in human studies. Several studies have found no overall increase in the risk of developing breast cancer. However, women who use oral contraceptives and have a strong family history of breast cancer or who have breast nodules or abnormal mammograms should be followed closely by their doctors. Some studies have reported an increase in the risk of developing breast cancer, particularly at a younger age. This increased risk appears to be related to duration of use.

Some studies have found an increase in the incidence of cancer of the cervix in women who use oral contraceptives. However, this finding may be related to factors other than the use of oral contraceptives.

ESTIMATED RISK OF DEATH FROM A BIRTH CONTROL METHOD OR PREGNANCY

All methods of birth control and pregnancy are associated with a risk of developing certain diseases which may lead to disability or death. An estimate of the number of deaths associated with different methods of birth control and pregnancy has been calculated and is shown in the following table:

ESTIMATED ANNUAL NUMBER OF BIRTH-RELATED OR METHOD-RELATED DEATHS ASSOCIATED WITH CONTROL OF FERTILITY PER 100,000 NON-STERILE WOMEN, BY FERTILITY CONTROL METHOD ACCORDING TO AGE

Method of control and outcome	15-19	20-24	25-29	30-34	35-39	40-44
No fertility control methods*	7.0	7.4	9.1	14.8	25.7	28.2
Oral contraceptives non-smoker**	0.3	0.5	0.9	1.9	13.8	31.6
Oral contraceptives smoker**	2.2	3.4	6.6	13.5	51.1	117.2
IUD**	0.8	0.8	1.0	1.0	1.4	1.4
Condom*	1.1	1.6	0.7	0.2	0.3	0.4
Diaphragm/Spermicide*	1.9	1.2	1.2	1.3	2.2	2.8
Periodic abstinence*	2.5	1.6	1.6	1.7	2.9	3.6

*Deaths are birth-related
**Deaths are method-related

In the above table, the risk of death from any birth control method is less than the risk of childbirth except for oral contraceptive users over the age of 35 who smoke and pill users over the age of 40 even if they do not smoke. It can be seen from the table that for women aged 15 to 39 the risk of death is highest with pregnancy (7–26 deaths per 100,000 women, depending on age). Among pill users who do not smoke the risk of death is always lower than that associated with pregnancy for any age group, although over the age of 40 the risk increases to 32 deaths per 100,000 women compared to 28 associated with pregnancy at that age. However, for pill users who smoke and are over the age of 35 the estimated number of deaths exceeds those for other methods of birth control. If a woman is over the age of 40 and smokes, her estimated risk of death is 4 times higher (117/100,000 women) than the estimated risk associated with pregnancy (28/100,000 women) in that age group.

The suggestion that women over 40 who don't smoke should not take oral contraceptives is based on information from older high-dose pills and on less selective use of pills than is practiced today. An Advisory Committee of the FDA discussed this issue in 1989 and recommended that the benefits of oral contraceptive use by healthy, non-smoking women over 40 years of age may outweigh the possible risks. However, all women, especially older women, are cautioned to use the lowest dose pill that is effective.

WARNING SIGNALS

If any of these adverse effects occur while you are taking oral contraceptives, call your doctor immediately:

- Sharp chest pain, coughing of blood or sudden shortness of breath (indicating a possible clot in the lung)
- Pain in the calf (indicating a possible clot in the leg)

lism) or eyes
- A history of blood clots in the deep veins of your legs
- Chest pain (angina pectoris)
- Known or suspected breast cancer or cancer of the lining of the uterus, cervix or vagina
- Unexplained vaginal bleeding (until a diagnosis is reached by your doctor)
- Yellowing of the whites of the eyes or of the skin (jaundice) during pregnancy or during previous use of the pill
- Liver tumor (benign or cancerous)
- Known or suspected pregnancy

Tell your health care provider if you have ever had any of these conditions. Your health care provider can recommend a safer method of birth control.

OTHER CONSIDERATIONS BEFORE TAKING ORAL CONTRACEPTIVES

Tell your health care provider if you have or have had:
- Breast nodules, fibrocystic disease of the breast, an abnormal breast x-ray or mammogram
- Diabetes
- Elevated cholesterol or triglycerides
- High blood pressure
- Migraine or other headaches or epilepsy
- Mental depression
- Gallbladder, heart or kidney disease
- History of scanty or irregular menstrual periods

Women with any of these conditions should be checked often by their health care provider if they choose to use oral contraceptives.

Also, be sure to inform your doctor or health care provider if you smoke or are on any medications.

RISKS OF TAKING ORAL CONTRACEPTIVES

1. Risk of developing blood clots

Blood clots and blockage of blood vessels are the most serious side effects of taking oral contraceptives. In particular, a clot in the legs can cause thrombophlebitis and a clot that travels to the lungs can cause a sudden blocking of the vessel carrying blood to the lungs. Rarely, clots occur in the blood vessels of the eye and may cause blindness, double vision, or impaired vision.

If you take oral contraceptives and need elective surgery, need to stay in bed for a prolonged illness or have recently delivered a baby, you may be at risk of developing blood clots. You should consult your doctor about stopping oral contraceptives three to four weeks before surgery and not taking oral contraceptives for two weeks after surgery or during bed rest. You should also not take oral contraceptives soon after delivery of a baby. It is advisable to wait for at least four weeks after delivery if you are not breast feeding. If you are breast feeding, you should wait until you have weaned your child before using the pill (see GENERAL PRECAUTIONS, While Breast Feeding).

2. Heart attacks and strokes

Oral contraceptives may increase the tendency to develop strokes (stoppage or rupture of blood vessels in the brain) and angina pectoris and heart attacks (blockage of blood vessels in the heart). Any of these conditions can cause death or temporary or permanent disability.

Smoking greatly increases the possibility of suffering heart attacks and strokes. Furthermore, smoking and the use of oral contraceptives greatly increase the chances of developing and dying of heart disease.

3. Gallbladder disease

Oral contraceptive users may have a greater risk than non-users of having gallbladder disease, although this risk may be related to pills containing high doses of estrogen.

4. Liver tumors

In rare cases, oral contraceptives can cause benign but dangerous liver tumors. These benign liver tumors can rupture and cause fatal internal bleeding. In addition, a possible but not definite association has been found with the pill and liver cancers in 2 studies in which a few women who developed these very rare cancers were found to have used oral contraceptives for long periods. However, liver cancers are extremely rare.

- Crushing chest pain or heaviness in the chest (indicating a possible heart attack)
- Sudden severe headache or vomiting, dizziness or fainting, disturbances of vision or speech, weakness or numbness in an arm or leg (indicating a possible stroke)
- Sudden partial or complete loss of vision (indicating a possible clot in the eye)
- Breast lumps (indicating possible breast cancer or fibrocystic disease of the breast: ask your doctor or health care provider to show you how to examine your breasts)
- Severe pain or tenderness in the stomach area (indicating a possible ruptured liver tumor)
- Difficulty in sleeping, weakness, lack of energy, fatigue or change in mood (possibly indicating severe depression)
- Jaundice or a yellowing of the skin or eyeballs, accompanied frequently by fever, fatigue, loss of appetite, dark colored urine or light colored bowel movements (indicating possible liver problems)

SIDE EFFECTS OF ORAL CONTRACEPTIVES

1. Vaginal bleeding

Irregular vaginal bleeding or spotting may occur while you are taking the pill. Irregular bleeding may vary from slight staining between menstrual periods to breakthrough bleeding which is a flow much like a regular period. Irregular bleeding occurs most often during the first few months of oral contraceptive use but may also occur after you have been taking the pill for some time. Such bleeding may be temporary and usually does not indicate any serious problem. It is important to continue taking your pills on schedule. If the bleeding occurs in more than 1 cycle or lasts for more than a few days, talk to your doctor or health care provider.

2. Contact lenses

If you wear contact lenses and notice a change in vision or an inability to wear your lenses, contact your doctor or health care provider.

3. Fluid retention

Oral contraceptives may cause edema (fluid retention) with swelling of the fingers or ankles and may raise your blood pressure. If you experience fluid retention, contact your doctor or health care provider.

4. Melasma (Mask of Pregnancy)

A spotty darkening of the skin is possible, particularly of the face.

5. Other side effects

Other side effects may include change in appetite, headache, nervousness, depression, dizziness, loss of scalp hair, rash and vaginal infections.

If any of these side effects occur, contact your doctor or health care provider.

GENERAL PRECAUTIONS

1. Missed periods and use of oral contraceptives before or during early pregnancy

At times you may not menstruate regularly after you have completed taking a cycle of pills. If you have taken your pills regularly and miss 1 menstrual period, continue taking your pills for the next cycle but be sure to inform your health care provider before doing so. If you have not taken the pills daily as instructed and miss 1 menstrual period, or if you miss 2 consecutive menstrual periods, you may be pregnant. You should stop taking oral contraceptives until you are sure you are not pregnant and continue to use another method of contraception.

There is no conclusive evidence that oral contraceptive use is associated with an increase in birth defects when taken inadvertently during early pregnancy. Previously, a few studies had reported that oral contraceptives might be associated with birth defects but these studies have not been confirmed. Nevertheless, oral contraceptives or any other drugs should not be used during pregnancy unless clearly necessary and prescribed by your doctor. You should check with your doctor about risks to your unborn child from any medication taken during pregnancy.

2. While breast feeding

If you are breast feeding, consult your doctor before starting oral contraceptives. Some of the drug will be passed on to the child in the milk. A few adverse effects on the child have been reported, including yellowing of the skin (jaundice) and breast enlargement. In addition, oral contraceptives may decrease the amount and quality of your milk. If possible, use another method of contraception while breast feeding. You should consider starting oral contraceptives only after you have weaned your child completely.

3. Laboratory tests

If you are scheduled for any laboratory tests, tell your doctor you are taking birth control pills. Certain blood tests may be affected by birth control pills.

4. Drug interactions

Certain drugs may interact with birth control pills to make them less effective in preventing pregnancy or cause an increase in breakthrough bleeding. Such drugs include rifampin; drugs used for epilepsy such as barbiturates (for example phenobarbital) and phenytoin (Dilantin is one brand of this drug); phenylbutazone (Butazolidin is one brand of this drug) and possibly certain antibiotics. You may need to use additional contraception when you take drugs which can make oral contraceptives less effective.

HOW TO TAKE ORAL CONTRACEPTIVES

1. General instructions

- You must take your pill every day according to the instructions. Oral contraceptives are most effective if taken no more than 24 hours apart. Take your pill at the same time every day so that you are less likely to forget to take it. You will then maintain the proper amount of drug in your body.
- If you are scheduled for surgery or you need prolonged bed rest you should advise your doctor that you are on the pill and stop taking the pill 4 weeks before surgery to avoid an increased risk of blood clots. It also is advisable not to start oral contraceptives sooner than 4 weeks after delivery of a baby.
- When you first begin to use the pill, you should use an additional method of protection until you have taken your first 7 pills.

Your physician has prescribed one of the following dosage schedules. Please follow the instructions appropriate for your schedule.

- 21-Day Schedule for BREVICON® (norethindrone and ethinyl estradiol), NORINYL® 1 + 35 (norethindrone and ethinyl estradiol), NORINYL® 1 + 50 (norethindrone and mestranol) Tablets: You may start taking the pill on Day 5 of your menstrual cycle or on Sunday. To start on Day 5, count the first day of menstrual flow as Day 1 and take the first pill on Day 5 of the menstrual cycle whether or not the flow has stopped. To start on Sunday, take the first pill on the first Sunday after your menstrual period begins. If it begins on Sunday, take the first pill that day. Whether you start on Day 5 or on Sunday, take another pill the same time each day, preferably at bedtime, for 21 days. Then wait for 7 days, during which time a menstrual period usually occurs, and begin taking 1 pill every day on the eighth day after you took your last pill, whether or not the menstrual flow has stopped. This cycle of 21 days on pills and 7 days off pills is repeated until the time for your visit with your physician or health care provider.
- 28-Day Schedule for BREVICON, NORINYL 1 + 35, NORINYL 1 + 50 Tablets: You may start taking the pill on Day 5 of your menstrual cycle or on Sunday. To start on Day 5, count the first day of menstrual flow as Day 1 and take the first white, yellow-green, or blue pill on Day 5 of the menstrual cycle whether or not the flow has stopped. To start on Sunday, take the first white, yellow-green, or blue pill on the first Sunday after your menstrual period begins. If it begins on Sunday, take the first pill that day. Whether you start on Day 5 or on Sunday, follow the sequence around the card for 21 days. Then take an orange pill from the bottom of the card each day for 7 days and expect a menstrual period during this week. The orange pills contain no active drug and are included simply for your convenience—to eliminate the need for counting days. After all 28 pills have been taken, whether bleeding has stopped or not, take the first white, yellow-green, or blue pill of the next cycle without any interruption. With the 28-day package, pills are taken every day with no gap between cycles until the time for your visit with your physician or health care provider.
- NOR-QD® (norethindrone) Tablets 0.35 mg Schedule: Take the first pill on the first day of the menstrual flow, and take another pill each day, every day until the time for your visit with your physician or health care provider. The pill should be taken at the same time of day, preferably at bedtime, and continued daily without interruption whether bleeding occurs or not. If prolonged bleeding occurs, you should consult your physician.
- 21-Day Schedule for TRI-NORINYL® (norethindrone and ethinyl estradiol) Tablets: Take the first blue pill on the first Sunday after your menstrual flow begins. If menstrual flow begins on Sunday, take the first blue pill on that day. Take 1 blue pill the same time each day, preferably at bedtime, for the first 7 days, 1 yellow-green pill daily for the next 9 days, and then 1 blue pill each day for 5 days. Wait for 7 days, during which time a menstrual period usually occurs, then begin a new cycle of pills on the eighth day after you took your last pill, whether or not the menstrual flow has stopped. This cycle of 21 days on pills and 7 days off pills is repeated until the time for your visit with your

---

tives, especially if you had irregular menstrual cycles before you used oral contraceptives. It may be advisable to postpone conception until you begin menstruating regularly once you have stopped taking the pill and desire pregnancy.

There does not appear to be any increase in birth defects in newborn babies when pregnancy occurs soon after stopping the pill.

6. Overdosage

Serious ill effects have not been reported following ingestion of large doses of oral contraceptives by young children. Overdosage may cause nausea and withdrawal bleeding in females. In case of overdosage, contact your health care provider or pharmacist.

7. Other information

Your health care provider will take a medical and family history and will examine you before prescribing oral contraceptives. You should be reexamined at least once a year. Be sure to inform your health care provider if there is a family history of any of the conditions listed previously in this leaflet. Be sure to keep all appointments with your health care provider because this is a time to determine if there are early signs of side effects from oral contraceptive use.

Do not use the drug for any condition other than the one for which it was prescribed. This drug has been prescribed specifically for you; do not give it to others who may want birth control pills.

If you want more information about birth control pills, ask your doctor or health care provider. They have a more technical leaflet called **PHYSICIAN LABELING** which you may wish to read.

NON-CONTRACEPTIVE HEALTH BENEFITS

In addition to preventing pregnancy, use of oral contraceptives may provide certain non-contraceptive health benefits:

- Menstrual cycles may become more regular
- Blood flow during menstruation may be lighter and less iron may be lost. Therefore, anemia due to iron deficiency is less likely to occur
- Pain or other symptoms during menstruation may be encountered less frequently
- Ectopic (tubal) pregnancy may occur less frequently
- Non-cancerous cysts or lumps in the breast may occur less frequently
- Acute pelvic inflammatory disease may occur less frequently
- Oral contraceptive use may provide some protection against developing two forms of cancer: cancer of the ovaries and cancer of the lining of the uterus

BRIEF SUMMARY
PATIENT PACKAGE INSERT

Oral contraceptives, also known as "birth control pills" or "the pill," are taken to prevent pregnancy and, when taken correctly, have a failure rate of about 1% per year when used without missing any pills. The typical failure rate of large numbers of pill users is less than 3% per year when women who miss pills are included. For most women, oral contraceptives are also free of serious or unpleasant side effects. However, forgetting to take oral contraceptives considerably increases the chances of pregnancy.

For the majority of women, oral contraceptives can be taken safely, but there are some women who are at high risk of developing certain serious diseases that can be life-threatening or may cause temporary or permanent disability. The risks associated with taking oral contraceptives increase significantly if you:

- Smoke
- Have high blood pressure, diabetes or high cholesterol
- Have or have had clotting disorders, heart attack, stroke, angina pectoris, cancer of the breast or sex organs, jaundice or malignant or benign liver tumors

You should not take the pill if you suspect you are pregnant or have unexplained vaginal bleeding.

Cigarette smoking increases the risk of serious cardiovascular side effects from oral contraceptive use. This risk increases with age and with heavy smoking (15 or more cigarettes per day) and is quite marked in women over 35 years of age. Women who use oral contraceptives are strongly advised not to smoke.

physician or health care provider.

- 28-Day Schedule for TRI-NORINYL Tablets: Take the first blue pill on the first Sunday after menstrual flow begins. If menstrual flow begins on Sunday, take the first blue pill on that day. Take 1 blue pill the same time each day, preferably at bedtime, for the first 7 days, 1 yellow-green pill daily for the next 9 days, and then 1 blue pill each day for 5 days. Take 1 orange pill daily for the next 7 days and expect a menstrual period during this week. The orange pills contain no active drug and are included simply for your convenience—to eliminate the need for counting days. After all 28 pills have been taken, whether bleeding has stopped or not, take the first blue pill of the next cycle without any interruption. With the 28-day package, a pill is taken every day with no gap between cycles until the time for your visit with your physician or health care provider.

2. Missed periods/breakthrough bleeding

At times, there may be no menstrual period after you complete a cycle of pills. If you miss 1 menstrual period but have taken the pills *exactly as you were supposed to,* continue as usual into the next cycle. If you have not taken the pills correctly, and have missed a menstrual period, *you may be pregnant* and you should stop taking oral contraceptives until your doctor determines whether or not you are pregnant. Until you can get to your doctor, use another form of contraception. If you miss 2 consecutive menstrual periods, you should stop taking the pills until it is determined that you are not pregnant.

Even if spotting or breakthrough bleeding should occur, continue the medication according to the schedule. Should spotting or breakthrough bleeding persist, you should notify your physician.

3. If you forget to take your pill

If you miss only 1 pill in a cycle, the chance of becoming pregnant is small. Take the missed pill as soon as you realize that you have forgotten it. Since the risk of pregnancy increases with each additional pill you skip, it is very important that you take each pill according to schedule.

If you miss 2 pills in a row, you should take 1 of the missed pills as soon as you remember, discard the other missed pill and take your regular pill for that day at the proper time. Furthermore, you should use an additional method of contraception in addition to taking your pills for the remainder of the cycle. If more than 2 pills in a row have been missed, discontinue taking your pills immediately and use an additional method of contraception until you have a period or your doctor determines that you are not pregnant. Missing orange pills in the 28-day schedule does not increase your chances of becoming pregnant.

4. Pregnancy due to pill failure

When taken correctly, the incidence of pill failure resulting in pregnancy is approximately 1% (i.e., 1 pregnancy per 100 women per year). If failure occurs, the risk to the fetus is minimal. The typical failure rate of large numbers of pill users is less than 3% when women who miss pills are included. If you become pregnant, you should discuss your pregnancy with your doctor.

5. Pregnancy after stopping the pill

There may be some delay in becoming pregnant after you stop using oral contracep-

Most side effects of the pill are not serious. The most common such effects are nausea, vomiting, bleeding between menstrual periods, weight gain, breast tenderness and difficulty wearing contact lenses. These side effects, especially nausea and vomiting, may subside within the first 3 months of use.

The serious side effects of the pill occur very infrequently, especially if you are in good health and are young. However, you should know that the following medical conditions have been associated with or made worse by the pill:

1. Blood clots in the legs (thrombophlebitis) or lungs (pulmonary embolism), stoppage or rupture of a blood vessel in the brain (stroke), blockage of blood vessels in the heart (heart attack or angina pectoris), eye or other organs of the body. As mentioned above, smoking increases the risk of heart attacks and strokes and subsequent serious medical consequences.
2. Liver tumors, which may rupture and cause severe bleeding. A possible but not definite association has been found with the pill and liver cancer. However, liver cancers are extremely rare.
3. High blood pressure, although blood pressure usually returns to normal when the pill is stopped.

The symptoms associated with these serious side effects are discussed in the detailed leaflet given to you with your supply of pills. Notify your doctor or health care provider if you notice any unusual physical disturbances while taking the pill. In addition, drugs such as rifampin, as well as some anti-convulsants and some antibiotics may decrease oral contraceptive effectiveness.

Studies to date of women taking the pill have not shown an increase in the incidence of cancer of the breast or cervix. There is, however, insufficient evidence to rule out the possibility that the pill may cause such cancers. Some studies have reported an increase in the risk of developing breast cancer, particularly at a younger age. This increased risk appears to be related to duration of use.

Taking the pill may provide some important non-contraceptive health benefits. These include less painful menstruation, less menstrual blood loss and anemia, fewer acute pelvic infections and fewer cancers of the ovary and the lining of the uterus.

Be sure to discuss any medical condition you may have with your health care provider. Your health care provider will take a medical and family history before prescribing oral contraceptives and will examine you. You should be reexamined at least once a year while taking oral contraceptives. The detailed patient information leaflet gives you further information which you should read and discuss with your health care provider.

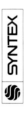 SYNTEX

SYNTEX (FP) INC.
HUMACAO, PR 00661

REVISED MARCH 1990
814-H2-218-90

© 1990 SYNTEX (FP) INC.

©1991 Syntex Laboratories, Inc.   pp. A-R and Appendix   Printed in U.S.A.   October 1991   CP92001   9118-58